Review Questions for Dentistry

Review Questions for Dentistry

Hugh Devlin

Professor of Restorative Dentistry,
University of Manchester,
Manchester, UK

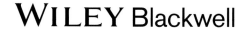

This edition first published 2017 © 2017 by John Wiley & Sons, Ltd

Registered office:
John Wiley & Sons, Ltd, The Atrium, Southern Gate, Chichester, West Sussex, PO19 8SQ, UK

Editorial offices:
9600 Garsington Road, Oxford, OX4 2DQ, UK
The Atrium, Southern Gate, Chichester, West Sussex, PO19 8SQ, UK
1606 Golden Aspen Drive, Suites 103 and 104, Ames, Iowa 50010, USA

For details of our global editorial offices, for customer services and for information about how to apply for permission to reuse the copyright material in this book please see our website at www.wiley.com/wiley-blackwell

The right of the author to be identified as the author of this work has been asserted in accordance with the UK Copyright, Designs and Patents Act 1988.

Library of Congress Cataloging-in-Publication Data

Names: Devlin, Hugh, 1954- , author.
Title: Review questions for dentistry / Hugh Devlin.
Description: Chichester, West Sussex ; Hoboken, NJ : John Wiley & Sons Inc.,
 2016. | Includes bibliographical references and index.
Identifiers: LCCN 2015042486 | ISBN 9781118815045 (pbk.)
Subjects: | MESH: Dentistry–Examination Questions. | Oral Surgical
 Procedures–Examination Questions.
Classification: LCC RK57 | NLM WU 18.2 | DDC 617.60076–dc23 LC record available at
 http://lccn.loc.gov/2015042486

A catalogue record for this book is available from the British Library.

Wiley also publishes its books in a variety of electronic formats. Some content that appears in print may not be available in electronic books.

Cover image ©Getty/GAnay Mutlu

Set in 9.5/13pt Meridien by SPi Global, Chennai, India

Printed in Singapore by C.O.S. Printers Pte Ltd

1   2017

Contents

About the companion website, vii

Introduction: How to approach answering multiple choice
   questions, ix

Section 1: Questions testing the introductory aspects of the subject

1 Endodontics, 3

2 Periodontology, 11

3 Operative dentistry, 19

4 Prosthodontics, 25

5 Medical and surgical aspects of oral and dental health, 33

6 Paediatric dentistry, public dental health and orthodontics, 40

Section 2: Questions exploring the subjects in more detail

7 Endodontics, 51

8 Periodontology, 75

9 Operative dentistry, 97

10 Prosthodontics, 118

11 Medical and surgical aspects of oral and dental health, 153

12 Paediatric dentistry, public dental health and orthodontics, 171

Further reading, 176

Index, 183

About the companion website

Review Questions for Dentistry is accompanied by a companion website:

www.wiley.com/go/devlin/review_questions_for_dentistry

The website includes:
- Interactive Multiple Choice Questions (MCQs)

Introduction

How to approach answering multiple choice questions

The primary purpose of any test question is to test your breadth and depth of knowledge about a subject. It may seem obvious, but reading the question carefully is mandatory. It takes time to understand what is being asked and then formulate the best response. While a particular answer may be factually correct, it may not be the best response to the question. I have also tested the application of knowledge whenever possible, so that it is not sufficient to only know a particular piece of information; the student has to appreciate how that information is used in clinical practice. I have divided the text into an introductory section and a later section which explores the subject in more detail.

An explanation of the correct answer is also added, using the best current research evidence. In the later sections, especially, supporting references are quoted. The introductory sections are suitable for preparation for the Bachelor of Dental Surgery degree, whereas the later sections have been prepared with higher examinations in mind, for example the Membership of the Joint Dental Faculties (MJDF) examination. The new format of Part 1 of the MJDF (from April 2016) will comprise 150 Single Best Answer Questions in a 3-hour examination. This book is intended to test a candidate's understanding of high-quality healthcare provision, which is also the main objective of the MJDF and the Overseas Registration Examination (ORE). At present, Part 1 of the ORE consists of Extended Matching Questions and Single Best Answer Questions.

I have used current curricula in various dental schools to develop as comprehensive a range as possible. Students have been involved in developing the questions, with their feedback being used to refine some questions. References are included to support the veracity of the correct answers whenever possible. I have varied the type and format of questions to avoid the reader becoming tired and bored with the same presentation of questions. Only one option is the correct answer, unless stated otherwise.

I hope to stimulate readers to read around the topics covered here. No one text can cover the huge variety of knowledge needed in the different disciplines of dentistry.

SECTION 1

Questions testing the introductory aspects of the subject

CHAPTER 1

Endodontics

Questions

1 The ideal position for the access cavity in anterior maxillary teeth should
   A conserve as much of the pulp chamber roof as possible
   B be positioned close to the incisal edge
   C be positioned over the cingulum of the tooth
   D be positioned to allow access to the apical region of the root canal
   E utilise any existing cervical labial restorations to avoid any further damage to the tooth

2 Choose the option which correctly completes this sentence. The working length can be defined as the distance from a reference point on the crown of the tooth
   A to the cemento-dentinal junction of the root apex or apical constriction
   B to the anatomic root apex
   C to a point about 2.5 mm short of the radiographic apex
   D to the enamel-dentine junction
   E to the radiographic apex

3 An apex locator is an electrical device which is used to measure the working length. This device works using
   A magnetic flux
   B electrical conductance
   C electrical Impedance

Review Questions for Dentistry, First Edition. Hugh Devlin.
© 2017 John Wiley & Sons, Ltd. Published 2017 by John Wiley & Sons, Ltd.
Companion Website: www.wiley.com/go/devlin/review_questions_for_dentistry

D light

E solar energy

4 A Gates-Glidden bur is used to prepare

A the apical third of a root canal

B the apical third of a root canal when it is particularly curved

C the access cavity

D the coronal two-thirds of the root canal

E the apical root canal when a file cannot be negotiated to the working length

5 During root canal treatment which description best describes the phenomenon of 'apical transportation of the root canal' or 'zipping'?

A Where the original shape of the root canal is preserved

B Where a strip perforation occurs near the coronal end of the canal

C An apical perforation

D A lateral perforation

E The file tends to straighten out during preparation of curved canals with uneven enlargement of the apical part of the canal

6 An initial 'glide pathway' in endodontics is created using

A rotary endodontic instruments

B anti-curvature filing

C frequent irrigation

D manual preparation to a no.10 ISO size file

E EDTA (ethylenediaminetetraacetic acid)

7 Temporary obturation of the access cavity may be necessary between appointments. Which is the material that provides the best seal?

A Coltosol F (Coltene Whaledent), which is a non-eugenol temporary filling material

B Fermit (Ivoclar vivadent), which is a resin-based material

C IRM (Caulk/Densply, USA), which is a reinforced zinc oxide/eugenol material

D Cotton wool with a 2 mm covering layer of Cavit temporary filling material

E Cotton wool plug

8 Complete the following sentence. The endodontic access cavity in an upper first molar is centred over

A the disto-occlusal aspect of the tooth

B the palato-occlusal aspect of the tooth

C the mesio-palatal cusp

D the mesio-occlusal aspect of the tooth

E any existing restorations to avoid further iatrogenic damage to the tooth

9 Various solutions have been used as endodontic irrigants. Which of the following solutions is the most cost-effective endodontic irrigant?

A 2.25% sodium hypochlorite

B 2% chlorhexidine

C Sterile saline

D Local anaesthetic solution

E Sterile water

10 The placement of a satisfactory root canal filling has been completed, but it is recommended to radiographically review the endodontic treatment to determine if healing has taken place. Complete the following sentence. Root canal treatment should be reassessed radiographically

A at 3 months after the initial treatment

B at 6 months after the initial treatment

C at 9 months after the initial treatment

D at 1 year after the initial treatment

E at 2 years after the initial treatment

11 Choose the option which correctly completes the following sentence.

In internal root resorption

A the typical appearance on a periapical radiograph involves an ovate, often symmetrical, widening of the root canal

B cone beam computerised tomography (CBCT) has no place in the diagnosis of these lesions due to the high radiation dose

C the affected teeth are painful in the early stages, and pain is often the presenting symptom

    D surgical endodontic therapy is the preferred treatment option in most cases

    E the lesion can be monitored as spontaneous repair can occur

12 What is the prevalence of a second canal in the mesiobuccal root of the permanent maxillary first molar?

    A Between 5 and 10% of these teeth

    B Between 11 and 20% of these teeth

    C Between 21 and 30% of these teeth

    D Between 30 and 40% of these teeth

    E Over 50% of these teeth

13 AH Plus® (Dentsply International) is a typical, modern endodontic sealer material. Choose the best option from the following statements which describe the properties of this material.

    A It has very good dimensional stability

    B It tends to discolour the tooth

    C It is radiolucent

    D It has poor tissue compatibility

    E It tends to release formaldehyde

14 Of the following options, the best definition of 'apexification' is that it

    A is normal development of the vital root

    B involves inducing a calcified wall at the apex of a non-vital tooth

    C is vital pulp treatment

    D is vital pulp treatment involving normal physiological root development

    E has the same definition as 'apexogenesis'

15 There is a small swelling in the labial sulcus associated with a carious, non-vital upper left central incisor. The swollen area and tooth are painful to touch. What is your diagnosis and immediate treatment?

Answers

1 *Correct answer D*: The ideal position of the access cavity is midway between the incisal edge and the cingulum, which will allow the least restricted access to the apical region of the root canal. A pre-operative radiograph is often helpful in obtaining the correct bur angulation. The access cavity should be smooth without any overhanging dentine.

2 *Correct answer A*: The cemento-dentinal junction (or apical constriction) is the ideal position for location of the apical reference point (see Pratten, D.H. and McDonald, N.J. Comparison of radiographic and electronic working lengths. *J. Endod.*, 1996, 22: 173–6). Electrical apex locators are being increasingly used as they provide a more accurate determination of the working length than radiographic methods. These instruments detect the apical constriction, which is the boundary between the pulpal and periodontal tissues. The location of the apical constriction varies between 0.5 and 2 mm from the radiographic apex.

Traditionally, the cemento-dentinal junction and the apical constriction have been thought of as being coincident; however, this is not always true (see Hassanien, E.E., Hashem, A. and Chalfin, H. Histomorphometric study of the root apex of mandibular premolar teeth: an attempt to correlate working length measured with electronic and radiograph methods to various anatomic positions in the apical portion of the canal. *J. Endod.*, 2008, **34**: 408–12). Extending root canal preparation to the apical constriction minimises any extrusion of infected debris into the apical periodontal tissues. However, the consequences of not removing any infected pulpal tissue between the coronal apical constriction and the cemento-dentinal junction have not been fully investigated.

3 *Correct answer C*: Apex locators measure the electrical impedance between the apical foramen and a reference electrode placed in the mouth.

4 *Correct answer D*: Gates-Glidden burs are onion-shaped burs of different sizes used to pre-flare the coronal two-thirds of the canal. To avoid lateral perforation of the root they have a blunt end and are used passively at low speed (about 2500 rpm).

5 *Correct answer E*

6 *Correct answer D*: A glide path is a prepared, a smooth channel that extends from the opening of the root canal in the pulp chamber to the apical constriction. Prior to using rotary endodontic files, the creation of an initial glide path to the working length with at least a size no. 10 hand file is essential. This can be performed using a size no. 10 stainless steel K-file which allows good tactile sensation. The rotary files then enlarge the width of the glide path to provide a continuously tapering canal. Anti-curvature filing is when the operator directs most of the force applied during filing away from the inner walls of curved root canals. This prevents a strip perforation of the thin inner walls.

Apical patency is a controversial technique which aims to create a smooth, debrided canal from the apical constriction to the canal orifice. Typically a size no. 10 Flexofile is passively introduced but if this encounters resistance, files of progressively smaller diameter (sizes 8 and 6) are used until the canal orifice is reached.

7 *Correct answer A*: Uçtaşli and Tinaz (2000) showed that a 3.5 mm thick layer of Coltosol provided a better endodontic seal than cements such as Fermit or IRM of similar thickness (Uçtaşli, M.B. and Tinaz, A.C. Microleakage of different types of temporary restorative materials used in endodontics. *J. Oral. Sci.*, 2000, 42: 63–7). However, this was an *in vitro* die penetration study and the materials were not tested under masticatory loading or thermal cycling. Webber *et al.* (1978) showed that a 3.5 mm layer of Cavit (3M ESPE) is necessary for effective sealing of the access cavity (Webber, R.T., del Rio, C.E., Brady, J.M. and Segall R.O. Sealing quality of a temporary filling material. *Oral. Surg. Oral. Med. Oral. Pathol.* 1978, Jul; **46(1):** 123–30).

8 *Correct answer D*

9 *Correct answer A*: Chlorhexidine solutions have been shown in some studies to have a similar bacteriocidal activity to sodium hypochlorite solutions; however, chlorhexidine is less effective at dissolving necrotic organic material. While water and saline solutions may be cheap, they are totally ineffective as bacteriocidal agents.

10 *Correct answer D*: According to the 'Quality guidelines for endodontic treatment: consensus report of the European Society of Endodontology' (see European Society of Endodontology. *Int. Endod. J.*, 2006, **39**: 921–30), the root canal treatment should be assessed after 1 year, and may need further follow-up for a minimum of 4 years if the prognosis seems uncertain. Assessment of endodontic success will also involve a clinical examination and detailed history taking. In particular, the presence of a sinus tract, and continued symptoms of pain and swelling indicate a failed treatment.

11 *Correct answer A*: cone beam computerised tomography (CBCT) provides a 3-D view of the root resorption and is often very useful in identifying whether the root has been perforated. In the early stages, internal root resorption is painless and vitality testing of the tooth often provides variable results that depend on the quantity of remaining vital pulp tissue present. Internal root resorption is often initiated by trauma which causes disruption of the odontoblast and predentine layers, allowing odontoclasts access to the dentine (see Wedenberg, C. and Lindskog, S. Evidence for a resorption inhibitor in dentine. *Eur. J. Oral. Sci.*, 1987, **95**: 205–11). Spontaneous repair of internal root resorption occurs very rarely, therefore active treatment is recommended.

12 *Correct answer E*: Several studies have shown that a second mesio-buccal canal (MB2) occurs in the majority of upper first molar teeth (see Peeters, H.H., Suardita, K. and Setijanto, D. Prevalence of a second canal in the mesiobuccal root of permanent maxillary first molars from an Indonesian population. *J. Oral. Sci.*, 2011, **53**: 489–94 and Wolcott, J., Ishley, D., Kennedy, W., Johnson, S. and Minnich, S. Clinical investigation of second mesiobuccal canals in endodontically treated and retreated maxillary molars. *J. Endod.*, 2002, **28**: 477–9).

13 *Correct answer A*: The composition of AH Plus® is based on an epoxide amine and other amines. It is self-adhesive and stable.

14 *Correct answer B*: Apexogenesis (not apexification) involves vital pulp treatment which encourages normal root development of the tooth.

15 *Correct answer*: The diagnosis is an acute apical abscess associated with an upper left central incisor tooth. The immediate treatment involves obtaining drainage of pus; if no fluctuant swelling is present then drain the abscess through the root canal by obtaining access through the tooth. If a fluctuant swelling is present then it is incised. If the patient has systemic symptoms of pyrexia then antibiotics should be considered.

CHAPTER 2

Periodontology

Questions

1 The Basic Periodontal Examination (BPE) uses a World Health Organisation probe with a black-coloured marking at 3.5 to 5.5 mm from the end of the probe. The gingival margin around the teeth (except the third molars) is probed and the highest score for each sextant recorded. A score of 3 for a sextant indicates that
   A furcation involvement is present
   B the probing depth around one of the teeth in that sextant is greater than 5.5 mm
   C the probing depth around one of the teeth in that sextant is between 3.5 and 5.5 mm
   D no calculus is present
   E bleeding has taken place following the probing

2 The prevalence of caries in the last 10 years in England has continued to decline. What is the proportion of the adult population that has severe periodontal disease (i.e. with at least one periodontal pocket greater than 6 mm)?
   A less than 10%
   B about 20%
   C about 30%
   D about 40%
   E about 50%

Review Questions for Dentistry, First Edition. Hugh Devlin.
© 2017 John Wiley & Sons, Ltd. Published 2017 by John Wiley & Sons, Ltd.
Companion Website: www.wiley.com/go/devlin/review_questions_for_dentistry

3 Which of the following medications does not induce gingival over-growth?
  A Ciclosporin (an immunosuppressant drug)
  B Oral contraceptive
  C Phenytoin (an anticonvulsant drug)
  D Aspirin
  E Nifedipine (a calcium channel blocker drug)

4 Probing of a gingival margin with a 25 g force is followed by bleed-ing. This usually indicates
  A that too great a force has been used
  B a gingival site that has more inflammation than a non-bleeding site
  C that the patient has serious disease, e.g. leukaemia
  D the patient smokes cigarettes
  E a diagnosis of chronic periodontitis

5 In treatment of periodontal disease, the principal aim of the 'initial phase of therapy' is to
  A establish a diagnosis
  B prevent recurrence of disease
  C restore aesthetics
  D carry out periodontal surgery
  E provide oral hygiene instruction and removal of plaque

6 Following a diagnosis of chronic periodontitis, where a patient has generalised 4 to 5 mm pocketing (BPE score = 3), root surface debridement is undertaken. When should the patient be recalled to assess the response to therapy and undertake detailed periodontal charting?
  A One week
  B Two weeks
  C Four to six weeks
  D Four months
  E Six months

7 What is the role of systemic antibiotics in the treatment of chronic periodontitis?
  A Systemic antibiotics can be used as an adjunct to root surface debridement

B Systemic antibiotics have no role in the treatment of chronic periodontitis

C Bacterial resistance is not a concern

D Allergic reactions are not a concern with systemic antibiotics

E The role of antibiotics is to eliminate all plaque bacteria

8 In the double retraction cord technique, gingival tissue retraction prior to impression taking for a crown allows the whole prepared tooth surface to be seen. Which statement is correct?

A The double retraction cord technique involves wrapping a single cord twice around the tooth

B An ultrathin cord (size 000) is initially placed in the gingival crevice followed by a slightly larger second cord which is removed just prior to taking the impression

C An ultrathin cord (size 000) is initially placed in the gingival crevice followed by a slightly larger second cord and both cords are removed prior to taking the impression

D An ultrathin cord (size 000) is initially placed in the gingival crevice followed by a slightly smaller second cord and both are removed prior to taking the impression

E Nowadays, all retraction cords are chemically impregnated

9 Which is the correct statement describing the effects of occlusal trauma?

A Trauma from the occlusion can initiate a periodontal pocket

B Temporary occlusal trauma on a tooth causes irreversible changes in the periodontium that prevent subsequent repair processes

C Traumatic occlusion can accentuate the loss of bone support associated with chronic periodontitis

D Occlusal trauma does not cause tooth movement

E Bone is not resorbed by excessive occlusal forces

10 Which of the following are risk factors for future periodontal disease?

A Tobacco smoking

B Diabetes

C Genetic factors

D Emotional stress
E All of the above

11 Which of the following statements is true?
  A Gingivitis always progresses to periodontitis
  B The progression of periodontitis commonly proceeds in a non-linear, episodic manner
  C Gingivitis and mild periodontitis are rare (seen in 5% of the population)
  D Chronic periodontitis is an inevitable result of ageing
  E Chronic periodontitis results from sub-gingival plaque containing gram-positive and aerobic organisms

12 Localised aggressive periodontitis is characterised by rapid progression of alveolar bone loss, but associated with low levels of plaque. Which of the following statements is correct?
  Localised aggressive periodontitis
  A has an onset at the menopause in women
  B is a common disease in Caucasians
  C does not have any link with a specific bacteria
  D can be treated with root surface instrumentation, surgical and antimicrobial treatments
  E is characterised by a weak serum antibody response

13 What is 'guided tissue regeneration'?

14 What is 'fremitus'?

15 What is the 'Miller index'?

Answers

1 *Correct answer C*

2 *Correct answer A*: The Adult Dental Health Survey (2009) showed that 9% of adults had severe periodontal disease. By comparison, nearly a third of dentate adults had clinically detectable dentinal caries (see White, D.A., Tsakos, G., Pitts, N.B. *et al.* Adult Dental Health Survey 2009: common oral health conditions and their impact on the population. *Br. Dent. J.*, 2012, **213**: 567–72).

3 *Correct answer D*: In rat models of drug-induced gingival overgrowth, pre-existing gingivitis is an important factor determining its severity (see Nishikawa, S., Nagata, T., Morisaki, I., Oka, T. and Ishida, H. Pathogenesis of drug-induced gingival overgrowth. A review of studies in the rat model. *J. Periodontol.*, 1996, **67**: 463–71).

4 *Correct answer B*: Patients who smoke generally have less frequent bleeding on probing. Bleeding on probing indicates an inflammation of the gingival pocket tissues; it does not indicate the patient has chronic periodontitis.

5 *Correct answer E*

6 *Correct answer C*: It is acceptable to recall the patient after an interval of four to six weeks, as a long junctional epithelial attachment would be expected to have formed by that time. A longer recall interval (e.g. 3 months) is needed when surgery has been undertaken. Where there is a poor response in some selected areas with substantial residual pocketing persisting, then periapical radiographs of the affected teeth may be needed to assist in their further assessment.

7 *Correct answer A*: The role of systemic antibiotics (such as amoxicillin and metronidazole) in the treatment of chronic periodontitis is controversial. The use of systemic metronidazole and amoxicillin has recently been found to be effective in some randomised clinical trials (see Feres, M., Soares, G.M., Mendes, J.A., Silva, M.P. *et al.* Metronidazole alone or with amoxicillin as adjuncts to non-surgical treatment of chronic periodontitis: a 1-year double-blinded, placebo-controlled, randomised clinical trial. *J. Clin. Periodont.*, 2012, **39**: 1149–58). Another study found a positive benefit for using systemic metronidazole in treating chronic periodontitis by reducing the number of residual pockets (see Preus, H.R., Gunleiksrud, T.M., Sandvik, L., Gjermo, P. and Baelum, V. A randomised, double-masked clinical trial comparing four periodontitis treatment strategies: 1-year clinical results. *J. Periodontol.*, 2013, **84**: 1075–86). Adjunctive systemic antibiotics may prove cost-effective by reducing the number of patients referred for further surgical procedures.

Mechanical debridement is an essential aspect of the treatment of chronic periodontal disease. However, in patients with moderate to advanced, progressive periodontal disease, a 1-week course of systemic metronidazole and amoxicillin (repeated every 4 months without additional measures) has been shown to arrest the progression of the disease (see López, N.J., Gamonal, J.A. and Martinez, B. Repeated metronidazole and amoxicillin treatment of periodontitis. A follow-up study. *J. Periodontol.*, 2000, **71**: 79–89). If further studies show that systemic antibiotics play a useful role, then their use will be in the elimination of periodontal pathogens (such as *P. gingivalis* and *P. intermedia*) and not the entire plaque biofilm. The effect of systemic antibiotics may be to kill bacteria in suspension, but the antibiotic resistance of bacteria in a biofilm may be much greater than when the same bacteria are free-floating. Bacteria on the bottom surface of the biofilm can invade the dentinal tubules making it difficult to remove them.

A recent study showed that 15% of patients had subgingival bacteria that were resistant to both amoxicillin and metronidazole (see Rams, T.E., Degenerm, J.E. and van Winkelhoff, A.J. Antibiotic resistance in human chronic periodontitis microbiota. *J. Periodontol.*, 2014, **85**: 160–9). Also, the patient must not be allergic to the prescribed antibiotic.

8 *Correct answer B*: The double cord technique is used when the sulcus is deeper as it provides greater displacement of the sulcus. Where the sulcus depth is 1.5 mm or less, the crown margins in the labial region of the anterior teeth should be placed about 0.5 mm below the gingival crest. This preserves the biological width below the restoration. Placement of a single ultrathin cord (size 000) during crown preparation allows gingival tissue retraction and accurate placement of the crown margin above the cord. A second, slightly larger retraction cord is placed in the region between the sulcus and the crown margin and removed just before impression taking.

9 *Correct answer C*

10 *Correct answer E*

11 *Correct answer B*: In chronic periodontitis, tissue damage is caused by the host response to bacterial plaque products crossing the junctional epithelium. Whereas the plaque bacteria initiate chronic periodontitis, the tissue destruction is the result of the host inflammatory response releasing enzymes (e.g. matrix metalloproteinases, prostaglandins, cytokines and interleukins). This response can be modified by environmental factors, such as smoking, and genetic factors, but it is not an inevitable result of ageing. Gingivitis and mild periodontitis are common and present in about 40–60% of the population. The sub-gingival plaque in periodontitis contains mainly a gram-negative, anaerobic complex of organisms. The effect of root surface instrumentation is to remove subgingival plaque, calculus and necrotic cementum with a resultant gain in attachment level and a reduction in the periodontal pocket depth.

12 *Correct answer D*: Localised aggressive periodontitis usually manifests at puberty. The rapid bone loss and tooth loss may be due to the inflammation that follows the strong antibody response to the initial infection with *Aggregatibacter actinomycetemcomitans*. Leukotoxin, secreted by *A. actinomycetemcomitans*, induces cell death amongst white blood cells (called apoptosis). This then allows the organism to further colonise the periodontal pocket.

13 *Correct answer*: Guided tissue regeneration is the regeneration of the periodontal attachment by the periodontal ligament cells following the exclusion of the gingival epithelial cells. Nyman *et al.* (1982) showed that a previously periodontitis-affected root surface does not prevent regeneration (Nyman, S., Lindhe, J., Karring, T. and Rylander, H. New attachment following surgical treatment of human periodontal disease. *J. Clin. Periodontol.,* 1982, **9:** 290–6).

14 *Correct answer:* Fremitus is a vibratory movement of the tooth that can be felt by palpating the tooth buccally when the patient is gently tapping their teeth up and down. A positive sign indicates occlusal trauma. Occlusal trauma can increase the rate of progression of pre-existing periodontal disease.

15 *Correct answer:* Miller's index has three classifications; class I describes a tooth moving up to 1 mm in a horizontal direction, class II when this horizontal movement is greater than 1 mm and class III when there is extreme horizontal and vertical movement.

CHAPTER 3

Operative dentistry

Questions

1 Vita classical (Lumin Vacuum) shade tabs can be used to choose the correct colour for a restoration. Which represents the correct ordering of the tabs in highest to lowest value (or brightness)?

A B1, A1, B2, D2, A2 and C1

B A1, A2, B1, B2, C1 and D2

C A1, B1, C1, A2, B2 and D2

D B1, B2, A1, D2, A2 and C1

E B1, A1, B2, A2, C1 and D2

2 A polycarboxylate cement is mixed and placed in a tooth as a temporary dressing. Which of these substances is not usually a constituent of the material during mixing?

A Water

B Zinc oxide

C Polyacylic acid

D Eugenol

E Magnesium oxide

3 High copper amalgams have improved corrosion resistant properties over conventional amalgam alloys. This is due to the

A presence of the silver-tin alloy

B the high content of the silver-mercury γ_1 phase

C the absence of the tin-mercury γ_2 phase

D absence of galvanic currents

E reduced plaque formation around high copper amalgam

Review Questions for Dentistry, First Edition. Hugh Devlin.
© 2017 John Wiley & Sons, Ltd. Published 2017 by John Wiley & Sons, Ltd.
Companion Website: www.wiley.com/go/devlin/review_questions_for_dentistry

4 Dental amalgam can undergo creep, resulting in marginal failure. What is creep?

   A The rigidity of a material

   B The time-dependent, permanent deformation under an applied load

   C The compressive strength of a material

   D The flexural strength of a material

   E Ductility

5 Which statement correctly completes the sentence? In a preventive resin restoration placed in a lower molar tooth

   A the fissures are routinely reduced to a depth of 1.5 mm

   B any carious dentine underlying the fissure is removed

   C any carious dentine underlying the fissure is usually sealed in place with a glass ionomer cement

   D any carious dentine can be treated with fluoride varnish

   E any carious dentine is removed and restored with amalgam

6 In cavity design classification, which option best completes the following sentence? A class V cavity is found on

   A the occlusal surface of a tooth

   B the interproximal surface of a tooth

   C the cervical third of the buccal or lingual surface of a tooth

   D the incisal edge of an anterior tooth

   E the fissures of a tooth

7 The Stephan curve illustrates the change in plaque pH over time following a rinse with a glucose drink. What is the 'critical pH' of enamel?

   A pH 2.5

   B pH 3.5

   C pH 4.5

   D pH 5.5

   E pH 6.5

8 What is tertiary dentine?

   A The dentine that is first deposited when the tooth is formed

   B Peritubular dentine

   C Intertubular dentine

D The zone of dentine under the carious lesion that is infected by bacteria

E Dentine produced by either odontoblasts or subodontoblastic progenitor cells in response to noxious stimuli

9 Computer-aided design/computer-assisted manufacture (CAD/CAM) techniques have been developed to produce milled ceramic inlays from optical impressions of the cavity. The following design features should be present in a mesio-occlusal (MO) cavity for a maxillary first premolar

A Rounded axio-pulpal line angle

B Minimum of 1.5–2 mm isthmus width to prevent fracture

C Rounded line angles

D 1.5 mm occlusal reduction

E All of the above features

10 Pins can be used to increase the retention of extensive amalgams. Which is the correct statement?

A A hole of minimum depth of 3 mm is made in the dentine

B Bending pins does not risk fracturing the dentine

C The self-threading pin is the least retentive type of pin

D A minimum of 1 mm of amalgam is necessary to cover the pin

E With larger diameter pins the retention of the amalgam is less

11 What is GV Black's (1836–1915) classification of carious lesions?

12 What is the procedure for the 'walking bleach technique'?

13 In preparing a tooth for a ceramic onlay, what is the minimum amount of cuspal reduction?

A 0.5 mm

B 1.0 mm

C 1.5 mm

D 2.0 mm

E 2.5 mm

14 Grooves placed in the interproximal box of a class II amalgam restoration should be

A positioned at the enamel-dentine junction

B positioned in the enamel

C positioned 0.5 mm deep to the enamel-dentine junction
D positioned 1.0 mm deep to the enamel-dentine junction
E positioned 1.5 mm deep to the enamel-dentine junction

15 In this cross-sectional diagram of a tooth with an occlusal amalgam, is the cavo-surface angle A or B?

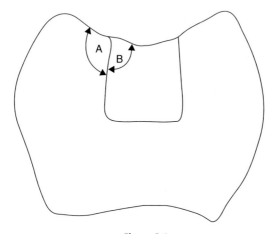

Figure 3.1

Answers

1 *Correct answer A*: The A shades are brownish, the B shades are yellowish, the C shades are greyish and the D shades are a brownish colour. The letter indicates the hue of the tab and the number the chroma.

2 *Correct answer D*

3 *Correct answer C*

4 *Correct answer B*

5 *Correct answer B*

6 *Correct answer C*: When the occlusal surface of a tooth has a cavity, it is classified as a class I cavity. When the interproximal surface of a molar tooth is affected, it is a class II cavity.

7 *Correct answer D*: The critical pH (5.5) is that acidity below which the enamel crystals of hydroxyapatite begin to dissociate. For dentine, the critical pH is 6.2, which explains why caries progress through dentine at a faster rate than enamel. Dentine caries can be extensive when there is a reduced salivary flow and buffering capacity, often due to drug therapy. The risk of further carious lesions developing can be reduced by recommending a high-concentration fluoride toothpaste, oral hygiene instruction, dietary advice, drinking water and chewing sugarless gum.

8 *Correct answer E*

9 *Correct answer E*

10 *Correct answer D*: A hole in dentine of length greater than 2 mm is unnecessary. With greater depth or number of pins, the danger of pulp penetration is increased.

11 *Correct answer*: Class I cavity: caries affecting the fissure or pit of an anterior or posterior tooth

Class II cavity: caries affecting the interproximal surface of a posterior (molar or premolar) tooth
Class III cavity: caries affecting the interproximal surface of an anterior tooth
Class IV cavity: caries affecting the interproximal surface and the incisal edge of an anterior tooth
Class V cavity: caries affecting the cervical third of an anterior or posterior tooth
Class VI cavity: caries affecting the cusp tip of a tooth

12 *Correct answer:* The gutta percha root filling is removed to 2 mm below the gingival margin. A thin layer of glass ionomer is placed over the gutta percha to prevent cervical root resorption. The access cavity is etched with 37% phosphoric acid, washed and dried. A pledget of cotton wool soaked in carbamide peroxide is sealed in the cavity with glass ionomer. The procedure is repeated twice at fortnightly intervals.

13 *Correct answer C:* In addition, the walls of the ceramic inlay preparation should be slightly divergent with rounded line angles and a chamfer finish line.

14 *Correct answer C:* The grooves should be directed laterally towards the buccal or lingual surface and not towards the pulp. The grooves prevent displacement of the amalgam.

15 *Correct answer A:* The cavosurface angle is the angle formed by the axial wall of the cavity with the external surface of the tooth.

CHAPTER 4

Prosthodontics

Questions

1 Which statement best completes the following sentence. A major advantage of an overdenture appliance is that
   A the abutment teeth are protected from caries
   B the abutment teeth are less prone to develop chronic periodontitis
   C the alveolar bone around the abutment teeth is preserved
   D the denture base over the abutment teeth is less prone to fracture
   E endodontic treatment of the abutment teeth is avoided

2 Which of the following factors does not predispose a patient to develop denture stomatitis?
   A Wearing complete dentures at night
   B Occlusal trauma
   C Poor denture hygiene
   D A diet rich in sucrose
   E Mandibular residual ridge reduction

3 Special trays (incorporating tissue stops) should be used for the definitive impression stage of partial dentures. What is the optimal thickness of spacing that should be designed when using an alginate impression material?
   A 0.5 mm
   B 1 mm
   C 2 mm
   D 3 mm
   E 4 mm

Review Questions for Dentistry, First Edition. Hugh Devlin.
© 2017 John Wiley & Sons, Ltd. Published 2017 by John Wiley & Sons, Ltd.
Companion Website: www.wiley.com/go/devlin/review_questions_for_dentistry

4 Which statement best completes the following sentence. Enamel erosion can be recognised clinically as

A a glossy appearance of the enamel surface

B cervical wear due to a damaging toothbrushing technique

C generalised gingival recession

D an increased caries rate

E a flat occlusal plane

5 Prior to sending impressions to the laboratory, they should be rinsed in running water and immersed in 1% sodium hypochlorite solution for 10 minutes. Once the disinfection is complete, the impressions are rinsed in water and sent to the laboratory in a sealed plastic bag. Which statement is correct?

A This disinfectant procedure can have harmful effects on the accuracy of the impression

B This disinfectant procedure has no harmful effects on the accuracy of the impression

C Alginate impressions do not imbibe water if left in the disinfectant solution for prolonged periods

D Alginate impression material is an example of a reversible hydrocolloid

E Alginate impression materials are accurate enough for crown and bridge materials

6 Choose the option which best completes the following sentence. A retainer is

A a part of the bridge that is luted to the abutment teeth

B a part of the bridge that replaces the missing tooth

C an abutment tooth

D a pontic

E a pier

7 In the construction of complete immediate dentures to replace upper and lower anterior teeth, which of the following difficulties may be encountered?

A Predicting the final shape of the residual ridge following tooth extraction

B Providing a stable occlusion in lateral excursions of the mandible

C Recording the retruded jaw relationship

D Obtaining the patient's approval of the trial denture aesthetics

E All of the above

8 The shortened dental arch (SDA) concept maintains a premolar and anterior tooth occlusion, without providing partial dentures to replace the missing molar teeth. In which of the following scenarios is the SDA concept most usefully employed?

  A When there are six natural lower anterior teeth opposing a complete denture

  B The patient is unable to maintain a healthy periodontal condition for their remaining teeth

  C The patient has a severe Class II Division 1 malocclusion with a large overjet

  D The patient's remaining teeth have active caries

  E The remaining anterior and premolar teeth have a good prognosis

9 What is the significance of the fovea palatinae in complete denture construction?

  A These midline landmarks provide a biometric guide to the position of the artificial posterior teeth on a complete denture

  B They indicate the most posterior extension of the upper impression tray

  C They are often relieved in the final denture

  D The fovea palatinae provide a guide to the correct positioning of the posterior palatal extension of the upper denture. It is usually adjacent to the 'vibrating line', which is the junction of the mobile soft palate and immobile hard palate

  E They form a hard bony region covered by mucoperiosteum, which is easily traumatised by the denture

10 What is the mean percentage of full metal crowns that survive after 10 years of service?

  A 95%

  B 68%

  C 48%

  D 20%

  E 10%

11 When constructing replacement complete dentures, the correct assessment of the patient's occlusal vertical dimension is essential. Which of the following options is correct?

A Freeway space is derived by subtracting the rest face height from the occlusal vertical dimension

B Freeway space is an equivalent term to occlusal vertical dimension

C Freeway space is derived by subtracting the occlusal vertical dimension from the rest face height

D Freeway space is measured using a Fox's occlusal plane guide

E Freeway space is assessed with the patient in a reclined position

12 Which of the following is not a risk factor for denture stomatitis in complete denture wearers?

A Poor denture hygiene

B Dentures that are poorly adapted to the underlying tissues

C Freeway space of 2–4 mm

D Occlusal trauma

E Continuous wearing of dentures over a prolonged period

13 What is the Kennedy classification for this partial denture?

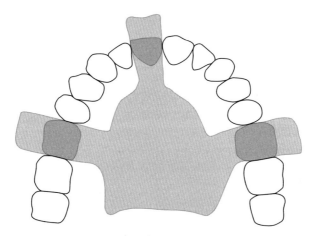

Figure 4.1

A Kennedy class I

B Kennedy class II

C Kennedy class III

D Kennedy class III mod 2

E Kennedy class IV

14 On what surface is the functional cusp bevel normally undertaken on a lower first molar crown preparation?

A The lingual inclined surface of the buccal cusp

B The buccal inclined surface of the lingual cusp

C The buccal inclined surface of the buccal cusp

D The lingual cusp

E None of the above

15 Why do we use the retruded jaw relationship when recording the jaw relationship in complete denture construction?

A It is a reproducible relationship between the upper and lower jaws

B It is a relationship that is routinely used when incising food

C It is easily recorded with a facebow record

D It can be easily recorded with a Willis bite gauge

E It can be easily recorded using a Fox occlusal plane guide

Answers

1 *Correct answer C*: A major advantage of overdenture treatment is that it preserves the alveolar bone and proprioception of the abutment teeth. However, a major disadvantage is that the abutment teeth are placed at increased risk of caries and periodontal disease. The denture base over the abutment teeth is often thin, making it prone to fracture.

2 *Correct answer E*: Residual ridge reduction is the progressive resorption of the bone surrounding the extraction socket. This may contribute to denture instability and denture trauma, but denture stomatitis is usually only observed to affect the palatal mucosal tissues under the upper denture. Patients should be encouraged to clean their dentures thoroughly with a brush and soap, and then leave them in water (or chlorhexidine solution) overnight. Miconazole cream can be applied to the fitting surface of the denture four times daily, but should be avoided in patients taking warfarin as it can increase their risk of bleeding.

3 *Correct answer D*

4 *Correct answer A*: Enamel erosion can be caused by a frequent consumption of acidic drinks. This causes a saucerisation of the incisal edges of teeth. On the posterior teeth, restorative filling materials are often left standing as 'islands' above the rest of the tooth. Attrition causes generalised tooth wear which results in a flat occlusal plane.

5 *Correct answer B*: Alginate is an irreversible hydrocolloid material (not a reversible hydrocolloid). In complete denture construction, alginate is the preferred material for impression taking when the patient has extensive bony undercut residual ridges. This is because alginate is an elastic material and removal of the impression will be more comfortable for the patient.

6 *Correct answer A*: A retainer is a part of the bridge that is luted to the abutment teeth, whereas the pontic replaces the missing tooth. An abutment is a tooth which supports a bridge. A pier is an abutment tooth that is located between the terminal abutments.

7 *Correct answer E*: If the patient has no posterior teeth, then recording a retruded contact position may be difficult as the patient
has postured forward during mastication for a number of years.
A canine-guided occlusion does not provide denture stability.
Placing upper incisors in the position of their natural predecessors
may not provide good aesthetics and the patient may object to the
change in tooth position as they are unable to view the anterior
tooth position prior to processing the denture. A try-in of the
upper anterior teeth is not possible before the teeth are extracted.

8 *Correct answer E*: The long-term success of the shortened dental
arch concept can only be guaranteed when the remaining teeth
have a good prognosis (i.e. no caries, abnormal toothwear or
chronic periodontitis are present). Where a large overjet is
present, the patient may only have a premolar occlusion. This
may cause an unsatisfactory masticatory function and a denture
may be preferred.

When there are only six natural lower anterior teeth present
opposing a complete upper denture, then this may cause tipping
movements of the denture during mastication. A lower partial
denture will provide a more even occlusion.

9 *Correct answer D*: The fovea palatinae are two small pits in the
soft palate which lie on either side of the midline. The upper
impression tray needs to be extended posterior to the fovea
palatinae; otherwise the processed denture will be underex-
tended. The posterior edge of the upper denture should lie along
the 'vibrating line' (which is the junction of the mobile soft
palate and immobile hard palate). The fovea palatinae provide a
guide to the correct positioning of the 'vibrating line'.

10 *Correct answer B*: Burke and Lucarotti (2009) showed that on average 68% of metal crowns were in service after 10 years (Burke,
F.J.T. and Lucarotti, P.S.K. Ten-year outcome of crowns placed
within the General Dental Services in England and Wales. *J. Dentistry*, 2009, **37**: 12–24). Bonded porcelain-metal crowns had a
less favourable survival (mean of 62% after 10 years). Only a
mean of 48% of porcelain crowns survived 10 years. Risk factors for crowns include endodontic treatment and tooth position,
with crowns on canine teeth having the poorest survival.

11 *Correct answer C*

12 *Correct answer C*: A freeway space of 2–4 mm is considered to be acceptable; it is measured using a Willis gauge.

13 *Correct answer D*: The Kennedy classification describes the number of edentulous saddles and whether these are free-ended or bounded. Free-end saddles have no distal abutment tooth, whereas bounded saddles have abutment teeth at either end.
Kennedy class I: describes a patient with bilateral free-end saddles
Kennedy class II: describes a patient with a unilateral free-end saddle
Kennedy class III: describes a patient with one bounded saddle
Kennedy class IV: describes a patient with an anterior bounded saddle which crosses the midline
   If a patient has one posterior bounded saddle and a free-end saddle, the denture classification is always based on the free-end saddle. Therefore, the denture in this case is classified as class II, but the additional bounded saddle is indicated as a modification, i.e. the complete classification is a class II mod 1 denture. Only class I, II and III dentures have modifications. A denture with three bounded posterior saddles would be a class III mod 2 denture.

14 *Correct answer C*

15 *Correct answer A*: If a flat surface is attached to the upper wax rim and a stylus to the lower rim, an arrow shape is produced, called a gothic arch tracing, when the patient moves their mandible to the left and right. The point of the arrow represents the retruded jaw relationship with the mandible in its unstrained relationship with the maxilla. Facebow recordings, the Willis bite gauge and the Fox occlusal plane guide cannot be used to record the retruded jaw relationship.

CHAPTER 5

Medical and surgical aspects of oral and dental health

Questions

1 How does a local anaesthetic cause temporary anaesthesia of the skin?
   A They prevent potassium ions entering the nerve cell
   B They prevent sodium ions entering the nerve cell
   C Local anaesthetic is a weak acid and is therefore lipid soluble
   D Large diameter fibres are most susceptible to local anaesthetic
   E The base form of the local anaesthetic is active inside the nerve

2 Midazolam, a short-acting benzodiazepine, is used widely for dental sedation. Which option best describes the method of action or properties of midazolam?
   A The benzodiazepines are receptor antagonists at the GABA/benzodiazepine receptor site in the central nervous system
   B Midazolam is metabolised in the liver to form potent metabolites which provide the majority of the biological activity
   C 100% of midazolam is absorbed when taken orally
   D Midazolam potentiates the inhibitory neurotransmitter gamma-aminobutyric acid (GABA) in the central nervous system
   E Midazolam is metabolised in the kidneys

Review Questions for Dentistry, First Edition. Hugh Devlin.
© 2017 John Wiley & Sons, Ltd. Published 2017 by John Wiley & Sons, Ltd.
Companion Website: www.wiley.com/go/devlin/review_questions_for_dentistry

3 In surgery, platelets assist in haemostasis by forming a plug in damaged blood vessels. Which of the following options is correct?

A Platelets contain a nucleus

B Platelets are about 20 μm in diameter

C Production of platelets is inhibited by thrombopoietin

D Platelets have a lifespan of about 60 days

E Platelets are formed in the bone marrow and are fragments of megakaryocyte cytoplasm

4 In the following diagram describing the coagulation phase of haemostasis, prothrombinase (factor Xa and cofactor FVa) activates 'A' converting it to thrombin. Thrombin acts on 'B' converting it to fibrin. What are 'A' and 'B'?

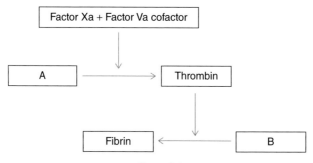

Figure 5.1

5 Anaemia is defined by the World Health Organisation (WHO) as

A Haemoglobin is less than 8 g/dl of blood in women

B Haemoglobin is less than 5 g/dl of blood in men

C Haemoglobin is less than 7 g/dl of blood in men

D Haemoglobin is less than 12 g/dl of blood in men

E Haemoglobin is less than 13g/dl of blood in men and less than 12 g/dl of blood in women

6 Midazolam is used for conscious intravenous (iv) sedation. Which of the following patients would be suitable for outpatient iv sedation?

A Patients categorised as American Society of Anesthesiologists grade ASA 1 and ASA 2

B A patient with heart failure

C A patient with renal failure undergoing dialysis

D A patient who is allergic to benzodiazepine

E Children with liver dysfunction

7 Von Willebrand's disease

   A affects only males

   B is caused by an absence of circulating fibrinogen

   C is caused by a low concentration or poorly functioning Von Willebrand factor in the blood

   D is the least common inherited bleeding disorder

   E always presents with severe symptoms

8 A patient consults you about a lump of soft tissue which has recently appeared on the attached gingiva between their upper central incisor teeth. The patient has no other significant medical history. On examination, the lump appears soft and bleeds easily on gentle probing. The adjacent teeth are vital. There is subgingival calculus present adjacent to the lesion. What is the most likely diagnosis?

9 A female patient returns with pain from an extraction socket three days after the uneventful extraction of a lower right first molar tooth. The patient has halitosis and a bad taste in their mouth. The patient smokes. On examination the socket appears to contain exposed bone but no healing tissue. What is the most likely diagnosis? How is the condition treated?

10 Which structures might be involved in a spreading infection that originates from the upper molar teeth?

   A The maxillary antrum

   B The soft palate

   C The hard palate

   D The pterygopalatine fossa

   E All of the above structures

11 Which option is correct? The mode of action of penicillin is to

   A inhibit protein synthesis in the bacterial cell

   B inhibit synthesis of deoxyribonucleic acid

   C act on the cell wall or membrane

   D inhibit mitochondrial enzymes

   E block binding of t-RNA

12 A dentigerous cyst

   A arises from the dental lamina at a very early stage of tooth development

   B is more common in females than males

   C may be detected fortuitously as a radiolucency that is associated with an impacted tooth

   D has a lining of ameloblast-like cells

   E most commonly affects the maxillary first molar tooth

13 What are the pre-operative radiographic features indicating that a mandibular third molar is in close proximity to the inferior alveolar nerve?

14 Which of the following are consistent features of a compound odontome?

   A Occur most commonly in the mandibular molar region

   B Appear as an irregular mass of calcified tissue

   C Contain 'denticles' or multiple, rudimentary teeth with enamel and dentine

   D Occur much more commonly in females

   E Can be left *in situ* as it rarely interferes with eruption of the permanent teeth, and never undergoes cystic change or bone resorption

15 Coronectomy is the removal of the crown of a mandibular third molar, rather than removing the whole tooth. The technique is especially useful where the tooth roots are in close proximity to the inferior alveolar nerve by avoiding damage to the nerve during surgery. Which of the following options is correct?

   A Following crown removal the pulp is removed and the canal obturated

   B The technique involves surgical separation of the roots and their gentle elevation from the socket

   C The technique is contraindicated when the lower third molar is non-vital

   D Following coronectomy, the roots do not migrate

   E Coronectomy may increase the incidence of injury to the inferior alveolar nerve

Answers

1 *Correct answer B*: Large diameter nerve fibres are less affected by local anaesthetics than smaller diameter fibres, with the result that the patient may be alarmed that they can experience pressure and touch sensation during a tooth extraction. The base form of the local anaesthetic diffuses through the nerve membrane into the nerve cell (pH about 6.5) where it ionises. The ionised form of local anaesthetics (not the base) is active inside the nerve where it blocks the sodium channels.

2 *Correct answer D*: Midazolam is poorly absorbed when given orally and is metabolised in the liver. Although active metabolites are formed when midazolam is metabolised, their effect is not clinically significant. Midazolam potentiates the inhibitory neurotransmitter gamma-aminobutyric acid (GABA) in the central nervous system. Flumazenil is a GABAA receptor antagonist and is used to treat those patients with a benzodiazepine overdose.

3 *Correct answer E*: Thrombopoietin stimulates production of platelets. Platelets do not have a nucleus, they have a lifespan of about 9–10 days and are about 2–4 μm in diameter.

4 *Correct answer*: A is prothrombin and B is fibrinogen.

5 *Correct answer E*

6 *Correct answer A*: Patients classed as ASA 1 and 2 are suitable for outpatient sedation. ASA 1 patients have no systemic disease. ASA 2 patients have systemic disease but it is well controlled and does not limit the patient's function. A patient with heart failure or who has renal failure treated by ongoing dialysis is classed as ASA 4, as this represents an ongoing, severe systemic disease that is life threatening. Midazolam is a water-soluble benzodiazepine, therefore patients who are allergic to benzodiazepines must not be given midazolam. In children, midazolam tends to cause disinhibition rather than sedation and it can also cause hallucinations (see Hosey, M.T. UK National Clinical Guidelines in Paediatric

Dentistry. Managing anxious children: the use of conscious sedation in paediatric dentistry. *Int. J. Paediatr. Dent.*, 2002, Sept; **12(5):** 359–72).

7 *Correct answer C*: In Von Willebrand's disease the symptoms can be mild and the condition can go unnoticed. It is the most common of the inherited bleeding disorders and can affect males or females.

8 *Correct answer*: Pyogenic granuloma. The differential diagnosis would be a fibrous epulis or peripheral giant cell granuloma.

9 *Correct answer*: Dry socket (alveolar osteitis). It is treated by gentle irrigation of the socket with 0.12% chlorhexidine and a dressing is applied containing Alvogyl™ paste. The patient should be reviewed in 2–3 days.The differential diagnosis would include a fractured mandible, osteonecrosis and osteomyelitis. Factors that predispose to dry socket include smoking, use of oral contraceptives, previous infection and a history of dry socket.

10 *Correct answer E*: The pterygopalatine fossa lies posterior to the maxilla and anterior to the pterygoid plates. The importance of clinical infection in this region is that it may spread to the orbital or cranial cavities.

11 *Correct answer C*

12 *Correct answer C*: The radiolucency is usually well-defined and unilocular (although it may appear to have a multilocular appearance occasionally). The follicle is enlarged and a dentigerous cyst is suspected if this space is greater than 3 mm on a radiograph. Cystic change begins after enamel formation has been completed, which is not an early stage of tooth development. The lining of a dentigerous cyst is usually composed of stratified squamous cells and is typically non-keratinised. Males are more commonly affected than females. The most commonly affected tooth is the mandibular third molar (see Lin, H.P., Wang, Y.P., Chen, H.M., Cheng, S.J., Sun, A. and Chiang, C.P. A clinicopathological study of 338 dentigerous cysts. *J. Oral. Pathol.* Med., 2013, **42(6):** 462–7).

13 *Correct answer*: These include:
1. Deflection of the roots of the third molar
2. A dark band present across the tooth root (may also be due to lingual cortical plate perforation)
3. Narrowing or deflection of the inferior alveolar canal
4. Loss over the tooth of the white opaque cortical border of the mandibular inferior alveolar nerve canal

14 *Correct answer C*: A compound odontome occurs most commonly in the anterior maxilla and often prevents eruption of the permanent teeth. Complex odontomes consist of an irregular mass of calcified tissue. The incidence of the compound odontome is slightly greater among males than females (see Yadav, M., Godge, P., Meghana, S.M. and Kulkarni, S.R. Compound odontoma. *Contemp. Clin. Dent.*, 2012, Apr; **3(Suppl 1):** S13–5).

15 *Correct answer C*: For a further discussion of the technique, see Renton, T., Hankins, M., Sproate, C. and McGurk, M. A randomised controlled clinical trial to compare the incidence of injury to the inferior alveolar nerve as a result of coronectomy and removal of mandibular third molars. *Br. J. Oral Maxillofac. Surg.*, 2005, Feb; **43(1):** 7–12).

CHAPTER 6

Paediatric dentistry, public dental health and orthodontics

Questions

1 The mineralisation of which teeth may be adversely affected by a mother's illness during pregnancy?
   A The permanent maxillary incisors
   B The permanent maxillary canines
   C The primary first molars
   D The permanent mandibular first premolars
   E The permanent mandibular central incisors

2 How does water fluoridation reduce the incidence of caries in children?
   Fluoride:
   A reduces the acidogenicity of plaque through an antimicrobial action
   B encourages re-mineralisation
   C inhibits demineralisation
   D forms fluorhydroxyapatite which is incorporated into the tooth surface making it more resistant to plaque acid
   E uses all of the above mechanisms

3 Which of the following conditions are **not** associated with non-carious tooth surface loss?
   A Gastro-oesophageal reflux
   B Eating disorders
   C Ruminating habits
   D Use of casein phosphopeptide-amorphous calcium phosphate (CPP-ACP) mousse
   E Aspirin use for the treatment of juvenile rheumatic arthritis

Review Questions for Dentistry, First Edition. Hugh Devlin.
© 2017 John Wiley & Sons, Ltd. Published 2017 by John Wiley & Sons, Ltd.
Companion Website: www.wiley.com/go/devlin/review_questions_for_dentistry

4 A young patient immediately attends your surgery following injury involving the pulp of a permanent incisor. You decide to undertake a pulpotomy. What cells will continue the growth of the root (labelled A) and what are the materials (C, D and E) that are applied to the tooth to encourage this apexogenesis? What occurs at the junction (labelled B) between the applied material and the pulp?

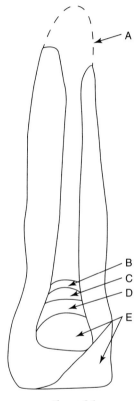

Figure 6.1

5 You identify a 10-year-old child with learning difficulties as having poor attendance, new anterior caries and multiple restorations in their teeth. What would you recommend in the future dental management of this patient?

A Fissure sealants should be applied to the pits and fissures of susceptible teeth

B A daily fluoride tablet (1 mg) should be sucked

C Fluoride varnish should be applied every 4 to 6 months
D Recommend the child brushes their teeth twice a day, spit out the toothpaste and avoid rinsing their mouth with water. Involve the carers in this
E Use all of the above methods

6 You perform an 'Index of Orthodontic Treatment Need' (IOTN) examination for a patient. The patient has an increased incisor overjet of 5 mm (3a) and an increased and complete overbite (3f). What Dental Health Component (DHC) of IOTN does this patient have?

7 In caries diagnosis for children, the frequency of bitewing radiograph examination is
A undertaken routinely every 2 or 3 years
B dependent on their caries risk
C dependent on the plaque score
D undertaken routinely if the patient is socially disadvantaged
E dependent on their salivary buffering capacity

8 In the serial extractions technique, originally described by Kjellgren in 1948, which teeth are extracted and what is the correct sequence?
A Primary canines, then first primary molars, and finally the first premolars
B Primary canines, then first primary molars, and finally second primary molars
C First primary molars, then second primary molars, and finally the first premolars
D Primary canines, then second primary molars, and finally first primary molars
E First primary molars, then primary canines, and finally the second primary molars

9 Cephalometry: The Frankfort plane is defined as the line between
A the anterior nasal spine and the posterior nasal spine
B the menton and the gonion
C the upper border of the external auditory meatus and the most inferior border of the bony margin of the orbit

D the middle of the sella turcica and the nasion

E the nasion and the menton

10 The best time to extract a lower first permanent molar of poor long-term prognosis that provides an optimum contact point between the second molar and premolar, is at

A about 7 years of age

B about 8.5 to 9.5 years of age

C about 10.5 to 11.5 years of age

D about 12 to 13.5 years of age

E about 14 to 14.5 years of age

11 Extraction of a carious lower left first primary molar may result in

A a balancing extraction of the upper left first primary molar

B a compensating extraction of the lower right first primary molar

C a shift in the lower centre line

D an increase in the upper incisor proclination

E a retroclination of the upper incisor teeth

12 A unilateral cleft lip

A is where the cleft is present on both sides of the lip

B is more common in women who smoke and drink alcohol in pregnancy

C is more common in girls

D occurs when the palatal shelves fail to fuse

E is usually closed at age 10 years

13 In obtaining consent for treatment for young people aged 16–17 years in the United Kingdom, which is the correct option?

A Young people of this age are capable of consenting to their own treatment, but their refusal of the treatment offered can be overridden by a person with parental responsibility or a court

B Young people of this age cannot be 'Gillick competent', therefore cannot consent to treatment

C The young person has to be 18 years of age to able to consent to treatment

D The young person is anxious and makes an unexpected decision, so this shows that they are not competent to consent to treatment

E Young people aged 16 lack capacity to consent to treatment

14 Which is the correct option?

    A The mesiodistal length of the deciduous canine and molars is usually less than that of the succeeding permanent canine and premolars

    B The 'ugly duckling' phase of tooth development occurs following eruption of the permanent canine teeth

    C A class 1 molar relationship exists when the mesio-buccal cusp of the lower first molar occludes with the buccal groove of the upper first molar

    D The permanent lower incisors usually develop in a position labial to the deciduous incisors

    E The mesiodistal length of the deciduous canine and molars is usually greater than that of the succeeding permanent canine and premolars, and the difference is called the 'leeway space'

15 Which is the correct option? As defined by the British Standard Institute classification, a class II division 1 malocclusion

    A has the molars in a class II relationship

    B has the lower incisor edges positioned anterior to the cingulum area of the upper incisors

    C usually has a decreased overjet

    D has the lower incisor edges positioned palatal to the cingulum of the upper incisors and there is an increased overjet

    E has retroclined upper incisors

Answers

1 *Correct answer C*: All of the primary teeth undergo mineralisation *in utero*, therefore at 21–24 months. Hypoplasia may result from maternal illness, maternal smoking or ingestion of excessive amounts of fluoride during pregnancy. Whether the child was born prematurely or was undernourished are also correlated with a high incidence of hypoplasia in primary teeth (see Needleman, H.L., Allred, E., Bellinger, D., Leviton, A., Rabinowitz, M. and Iverson, K. Antecedents and correlates of hypoplastic enamel defects of primary incisors. *Pediatr. Dent.*, 1992, **14(3):** 158–66). The permanent central incisors begin to calcify at 3–4 months after birth, the permanent maxillary canines at 4–5 months and the permanent mandibular first premolars at 21–24 months.

2 *Correct answer E*

3 *Correct answer D*: Gastro-oesophageal reflux, eating disorders, use of aspirin for chronic painful conditions and ruminating habits are associated with erosion of teeth. Casein phosphopeptide-amorphous calcium phosphate (CPP-ACP) can remineralise teeth.

4 *Correct answer*:
   A is the Hertwig's root sheath
   B is a calcified barrier
   C is a non-setting calcium hydroxide
   D is a glass ionomer cement
   E is a resin composite restoration
   The figure illustrates a partial pulpotomy for a vital permanent tooth. Avoid a blood clot between the pulpal tissue and calcium hydroxide. Mineral trioxide aggregate may be used instead of calcium hydroxide. If the tooth is non-vital, then the pulpal contents are instrumented to within 1 mm of the radiographic apex and the canal is irrigated with a 1% sodium hypochlorite solution. The root canal is obturated with a non-setting calcium hydroxide dressing, which is replaced at regular intervals until a calcified barrier is formed.

5 *Correct answer E*: This child is at high risk of further caries. Dietary advice to carers and the patient are essential. The toothpaste used should contain at least 1000 ppm fluoride. The amount and frequency of sugar consumption between meals should be reduced. Any barriers to the patient's attendance should be explored with the carers, and attendance encouraged. The dentist should be aware of other factors that increase a patient's caries risk, for example wearing an orthodontic appliance.

6 *Correct answer 3a*: The IOTN examination is graded according to a hierarchy with overjet assuming more importance in this classification than crossbite, crowding or overbite.

7 *Correct answer B*: The risk of future caries in children is dependent on many factors (salivary buffering capacity, social disadvantage and plaque score), but the most important is their previous caries experience. It is currently recommended that children with high caries risk receive six-monthly bitewing radiographs, those with moderate caries risk receive annual bitewing radiographs and those at low risk of caries receive bitewing radiographs at 12–18 month intervals. The European Academy of Paediatric Dentistry recommend bitewing radiography is considered for all 5-year-old children, when they reach the age of 8–9 years and again at 12–14 years. There is likely to be further research and discussion in the future which clarifies the advice to dentists.

8 *Correct answer A*: The serial extraction technique begins with the extraction of the primary canines at about age 9 years in children with a class I malocclusion. This relieves crowding of the permanent incisor teeth. This is followed at about age 10 years with the extraction of the primary first molars. When the permanent canines start to erupt, the first premolars are extracted.

9 *Correct answer C*: The maxillary plane is defined as the line joining the anterior nasal spine and the posterior nasal spine. It normally forms an angle of $109° \pm 6°$ with the long axis of the upper central incisor tooth. The line joining the menton and gonion forms the mandibular plane. The line joining the sella turcica and the nasion is an approximation to the anterior cranial base.

10 *Correct answer B*: The best time to extract the lower first permanent molar is at age 8.5 to 9.5 years when the furcal bifurcation of the lower second molar is calcifying.

11 *Correct answer C*: In this situation, a balancing extraction would be the removal of a lower right primary molar. A compensating extraction involves the removal of an upper left first primary molar. The extraction of a lower left first primary molar may result in a centre line shift, but the likelihood of this occurring depends on the degree of crowding present.

12 *Correct answer B*: A cleft lip is more common in boys. A cleft lip is usually closed surgically in the first two to three months after birth.

13 *Correct answer A*: A young person is 'Gillick competent' if they have sufficient understanding and maturity to understand the advantages and disadvantages of a procedure and therefore give true consent. If patients are anxious then further careful explanation may be needed; the dentist cannot conclude that they are not capable of giving consent.

14 *Correct answer E*: The 'ugly duckling' phase of tooth development occurs prior to eruption of the permanent canine teeth. The incisors are spaced. The crowns of the lateral incisors are tilted labially. A class 1 molar relationship exists when the mesio-buccal cusp of the upper first molar occludes with the buccal groove of the lower first molar.

15 *Correct answer D*: The British Standard Institute classification is based on the incisor, and not the molar, relationship.

Questions exploring the subjects in more detail

CHAPTER 7

Endodontics

Questions

1 Inflammation of the pulp is often caused by
  A the toxic effects of dental materials
  B bacterial toxins diffusing from the carious cavity to the pulp
  C blood-borne bacteria
  D etching of dentin with 37% phosphoric acid
  E high speed carbide bur preparation rather than low speed bur preparation

2 After cavity preparation and placement of a large amalgam restoration, a patient experiences thermal symptoms.
  A The pulp should have been protected with a 2 mm thick base material
  B The patient's symptoms are usually very mild and short-lived
  C The pulpal nerves are unlikely to be responding to fluid movements in the dentinal tubules
  D Modern theory now holds that the marginal seal of restorations is of secondary importance
  E Copal varnish should have been used, as it provides thermal insulation

3 In a traditional access cavity for an upper maxillary first molar undergoing endodontic treatment
  A the cavities should be restored with acid-etch retained resin-composite restorations in preference to amalgam

Review Questions for Dentistry, First Edition. Hugh Devlin.
© 2017 John Wiley & Sons, Ltd. Published 2017 by John Wiley & Sons, Ltd.
Companion Website: www.wiley.com/go/devlin/review_questions_for_dentistry

    B glass ionomer as a liner does not reduce the contraction of resin-composite restorations

    C the main mesio-buccal canal orifice (MB-1) is usually positioned palatal to the distobuccal orifice

    D only a small part of the roof of the pulp chamber needs to be removed

    E removing the coronal dentine has no effect on the tooth's fracture resistance

4 Crown-down technique

    A is recommended for treating infected dilacerated and other curved root canals

    B is a serial instrumentation technique which uses successively larger instruments used in a reaming action

    C does not usually involve the use of nickel-titanium rotary files

    D is associated with a high failure rate

    E involves removal of the canal contents from the apical working length towards the canal orifice

5 The balanced force technique

    A is recommended for treating infected curved root canals because there is less likelihood of an 'apical zip'

    B if used properly negates the need for hypochlorite irrigation

    C does not remove dentine from the root canal wall

    D involves circumferential filing in a clockwise direction

    E involves the use of stiff files

6 Preparation of the root canal with a file

    A allows access of a disinfecting irrigant and so reduces the bacterial count

    B eliminates bacteria that have penetrated into the apical dentine

    C eradicates debris from any irregularly shaped root canal

    D can overlook any subsequent requirements for post preparation

    E may leave 0.25 mm of dentine wall thickness

7 An access cavity to the root canal system in the tooth

    A usually also involves removing existing defective restorations and caries first

    B always require that rubber dam be placed first of all

    C should usually be undercut to retain a temporary restoration

    D does not usually provide straight line access to the apical region

    E is positioned dependent only on the tooth's occlusal anatomy

8 Between appointment endodontic 'flare-up' emergencies

    A occur in about 25% of cases

    B are more prevalent in those with no history of pre-operative pain

    C are associated with a poorer success rate than those patients where no flare-up occurs

    D are more prevalent in those with pre-operative symptoms

    E are more prevalent in those with diabetes mellitus

9 The root canal irrigant, sodium hypochlorite

    A dissolves necrotic pulp tissue

    B is usually used at a 10% concentration

    C is acidic with a pH of about 5

    D does not affect the dentine, even with prolonged contact

    E possesses a narrow spectrum antimicrobial activity

10 One of the main distinguishing characteristics between a tooth affected by acute periapical periodontitis and one with chronic periodontitis is that

    A in chronic periodontitis the tooth is usually vital

    B in acute periapical periodontitis the tooth is usually vital

    C in acute periapical periodontitis the pain is poorly localised with applied pressure

    D in chronic periodontitis, only adults are affected

    E in acute periapical periodontitis the disease is classified as either localised or generalised disease

11 A patient has a tooth with a periodontal lesion in association with an endodontic lesion. Which statement is correct?

    A The periodontal lesion should be treated and controlled first

    B The endodontic lesion should be treated and controlled first

    C The tooth should be extracted as it will have a hopeless prognosis

D The periapical bone loss results from the periodontal component

E This arises from the bacterial invasion of dentinal tubules following root surface debridement

12 A regenerative endodontic procedure in an incisor with an open apex involves the induction of new dentine formation on the root canal wall and continued root development. To ensure continued treatment success of the regenerative procedure, the most important factor from the following options is

A to eliminate any infection

B to obtain informed consent from the patient

C to obtain revascularisation of the pulpal tissues using calcium hydroxide dressings replaced over a six month period

D to avoid forming a blood clot

E to avoid using mineral trioxide aggregate

13 Which of the following mechanisms protect the pulp when caries is advancing through the dentine?

A Components of saliva cause mineral deposition in the lesion

B The production of tertiary dentine

C The production of secondary dentine

D The production of primary dentine

E The production of mantle dentine

14 Stages in undertaking root canal treatment.

Place the most appropriate terms below in the correct position in the text

A Access cavity

B Filling with gutta percha

C Apical preparation

D Estimation of the working length

E Locate the canal orifices

F Restoration

G Coronal flaring

When suitable radiographs have been taken and an endodontic procedure is planned, the proposed procedure with its possible adverse effects and any alternative treatments are explained to the patient. The first stage in endodontics is to obtain an _____ and thereby _____. Any damage to the pulpal floor is avoided, but the roof of the pulp chamber must be removed. _____ removes the bulk of infected coronal tissue and prevents it from being carried into the apical tissues. Apex locating devices can be used for _____. The step-back technique involves a method of _____ such that accurate adaptation and _____ is enabled. Finally, the access cavity is restored.

15 Root perforations repaired with either a surgical or combined surgical and non-surgical approach have the worst success rate where the perforation is
A located at the osseous crest
B located at the apex
C located at the apical third
D located at the middle third of the root
E located in the mandibular teeth

16 Rotary file separation during the cleaning of a root canal can be prevented by
A watching for wear of the rotary file
B avoiding coronal flaring
C keeping the rotary file in the canal for as short a time as possible
D using steady pressure on the file when resistance is first encountered
E using the rotary file in a pecking action

17 A lower first molar has a small periapical inflammatory lesion limited to the cancellous bone. Which imaging technique would have the highest sensitivity in identifying the lesion?
A Dental panoramic radiograph
B Cone-beam computed tomography
C Mandibular true occlusal radiograph
D Periapical radiography
E All of the above are equally sensitive

18 When should a root filling be assessed radiographically to determine if the treatment is successful?
A Radiography is not used as the diagnosis of success if based on the absence of clinical symptoms
B At 5 years after completion of the root filling
C At annual intervals until 5 years after completion of the root filling

D Immediately after root canal treatment is completed, at 1 year after treatment and subsequently as required up to 4 years

E At 10 years after completion of the root filling

19 K-flex files are a type of hand file used in preparing the root canal to the correct shape and taper. In cross-section this file

A is diamond or rhomboid in cross-section

B is triangular in cross-section

C is circular in cross-section

D is rectangular in cross-section

E is oval in cross-section

20 One anatomical reason for the difficulty in anaesthetising mandibular teeth is that there can be accessory retromolar foraminae with innervation from the long buccal nerve or branches of the inferior alveolar nerve prior to its entering the mandible. What is the approximate incidence of these substantial retromolar foraminae?

A 0.6%

B 15%

C 35%

D 46%

E 60%

21 In the Gow-Gates technique, the point of entry of the needle is

A midway between the internal oblique ridge and the pterygo-mandibular raphe

B lateral to the external oblique ridge

C medial to the pterygo-mandibular raphe

D at the same height as the conventional technique, about 1 cm above the mandibular occlusal plane

E through the pterygo-mandibular raphe

22 When considering whether a prepared root canal can be obturated following placement of an inter-appointment dressing, which of the following statements are true?

A The tooth must not be associated with a fistula

B The tooth must be symptom-free

C The root canal can be slightly moist

D Microbiological testing is usually advised

E The root canal space must be free of all bacteria

23 Ledermix paste (manufactured by Sigma Pharmaceuticals Pty Ltd.) is used to reduce the pain associated with acute pulpitis. Which of the following form one of its active ingredients?

A Triamcinolone acetonitride

B Amoxycillin

C Penicillin

D Metronidazole

E EDTA (Ethylenediaminetetraacetic acid)

24 Cone beam computed tomography (CBCT) has transformed endodontic diagnosis. Which of the following statements is correct?

A Metal posts do not cause beam hardening or scatter artefacts in CBCT

B The effective dose using CBCT is less than that from a panoramic radiograph

C CBCT can produce a 3-D image of the teeth, displaying it simultaneously in axial, sagittal and coronal anatomical planes

D The CBCT image magnification is not the same in the different anatomical planes

E Capture of small volumes of data around a few teeth is not possible

25 Describe the properties of recently developed nickel titanium rotary files.

26 When should a coronal restoration be placed after root canal treatment?

A As soon as possible after completion of root canal treatment

B At 6 months, when apical bone healing has usually taken place

C At 12 months, when the likely success of the endodontic treatment is known

D At 18 months

E At 2 years

27 Pathological root resorption can be caused by trauma and pulpal infection. Which of the following systemic conditions is not related to root resorption?

A Hyperparathyroidism

B Osteoporosis

C Paget's disease

D Kidney disease

E Papillon–Lefèvre syndrome

28 What is the principal component of mineral trioxide aggregate?

A Calcium hydroxide

B Chlorhexidine

C Iodine

D Calcium silicate

E Bismuth oxide

29 As a result of toothwear, the pulp chamber may be seen to be obliterated on radiographs. What process causes this?

A Deposition of secondary dentine

B Deposition of reactionary dentine in the pulp horns

C Deposition of reactionary dentine on the floor and roof of the pulp chamber

D A thickening of the root dentine

E It is a normal ageing process

30 When assessing a tooth to determine whether endodontic is a suitable treatment option, which of the following does NOT contraindicate endodontic treatment?

A Extensive subgingival caries

B The dentist lacks the necessary endodontic skills

C The patient's attitude is unreceptive and unwilling to accept endodontic treatment

D The tooth forms an abutment of a bridge

E An inability to gain access to within 0.5 mm of the radiographic apex

31 The Thermafil® obturation system (manufactured by Dentsply Tulsa Dental Specialities) uses

A a heat plugger is used to soften the master gutta percha cone. The cone is then compacted into place using pluggers

B heated gutta percha is injected into the canal and then compacted into place

C cold lateral condensation of gutta percha

D flexible plastic rods covered with 'alpha phase' gutta percha,
   which are heated and then placed in the root canal

E thermomechanical compaction

32 A ledge has been created during instrumentation of the canal.
   What is the best way of managing this complication?

   A Periradicular surgery

   B Pre-curving the apical few millimetres of the file and using
      the modified tip to find the original canal path. This is then
      enlarged to regain access to the apical region

   C Sustained apical pressure on the file to force it past the ledge

   D Sustained apical pressure with the use of canal lubricants

   E Using irrigation to remove compacted debris

33 A working length radiograph is obtained

   A after gaining access to the pulp chamber and coronal prepara-
      tion has been carried out

   B after gaining access to the pulp chamber

   C after apical preparation has been completed

   D after rubber dam placement

   E pre-operatively

34 Describe the 'step-down technique'.

35 Correctly identifying the position for coronal access to the root
   canals can often be challenging. Which technique would you
   advise for locating the position of the second mesio-buccal (mb2)
   canal of an upper first molar tooth?

   A Plentiful irrigation with sodium hypochlorite solution

   B Parallax radiographic views

   C The second mesiobuccal (mb2) canal usually lies on a line
      between the palatal canal and the first mesiobuccal canal
      (mb1). The mb2 canal is located at the intersection of a per-
      pendicular line drawn between this line and the distobuccal
      canal

D Using a Canal Finder (Endotechnic, San Diego, USA)

E Widen access to the the mb1 canal, as the mb1 and mb2 canals frequently merge together

36 What is the 'inside-out' bleaching technique?

37 Fibre posts for restoring endodontically treated teeth can be classified into carbon, glass, or quartz fibre posts. What is the most common reason reported for clinical failure of luted fibre posts?

A Post debonding with loss of retention

B Fracture of the root

C Poor aesthetics due to water absorption

D Periodontal disease

E Fracture of the post

38 A separated endodontic file can prevent satisfactory disinfection and obturation of a root canal. Which of the following would not be included in the first line of treatment in removing a file that had fractured in the middle third of a straight root?

A Taking a radiograph to confirm the separation of the file and its position

B Attempt to remove the file with an endosonic tip

C Using small files to remove or bypass the separated file

D Surgical removal of the separated file

E Explain to the patient in a factual manner what had occurred

39 A small apical radiolucency is observed on a periapical radiograph of an upper central incisor tooth. The patient has complained of pain for a few weeks. Which of the following causes direct bone resorption in this situation?

A Macrophages

B Lymphocytes

C Mixed bacterial flora

D Granuloma formation

E Osteoclasts

40 In the diagram below, the apical region of the tooth has been altered by the straightening of the stiff file during root canal preparation. The shaded area in grey has been removed inadvertently. Give the names of the regions labelled A and B.

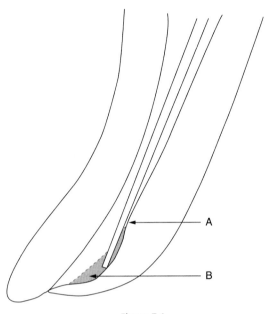

A

B

Figure 7.1

Answers

1 *Correct answer B*: 'Anachoresis' or the blood-borne spread of bacteria, as a cause of asymptomatic periapical or pulpal disease is unlikely. Fukushima *et al.* (1990) examined previously endodontically obturated teeth with asymptomatic apical pathology and found that a bacterial biofilm was present in the root canal, but not on the surface of the root. They concluded that the infection was introduced before or during endodontic treatment. (Fukushima, H., Yamamoto, K., Hirohata, K., Sagawa, H., Leung, K.P. and Walker, C.B. Localization and identification of root canal bacteria in clinically asymptomatic periapical pathosis. *J. Endod.*, 1990, **16**: 534–8). Animal experiments have shown that root canals that have been instrumented but left unfilled do not contain test organisms injected intravenously (Delivanis, P.D., Snowden, R.B. and Doyle, R.J. Localization of blood-borne bacteria in instrumented unfilled root canals. *Oral Surg. Oral. Med. Oral Pathol.*, 1981, **52**: 430–2). The main organisms present in persistent endodontic infections are facultative anaerobic and obligate anaerobic bacteria, organisms that would be expected to survive well in the root canal system.

There is an infrequent prevalence of an extra-radicular biofilm in some teeth where its location prevents access of disinfectant solutions and files to the bacteria. In those affected cases, an extra-radicular biofilm may inhibit effective treatment. This may result in 5–15% of teeth developing post-treatment apical periodontitis despite an adequate standard of care. In a study by Ricucci *et al.* (2009) of 12 symptomatic and 12 asymptomatic patients, bacterial infection of the periradicular space was always associated with bacteria in the root canal system (Ricucci, D., Siqueira, J.F. Jr, Bate, A.L. and Pitt Ford, T.R. Histologic investigation of root canal-treated teeth with apical periodontitis: a retrospective study from twenty-four patients. *J. Endod.*, 2009, **35**: 493–502). There is no evidence that an extra-radicular infection can exist without an intra-radicular infection also being present.

The use of high, rather than low speed, tooth preparation does not result in pulpal inflammation, provided that adequate water coolant is used. Modern endodontic filling materials and sealants are biocompatible, therefore extrusion of these materials is unlikely to cause more than a transient tissue injury. Post treatment disease is more likely to be related to the poor apical seal and an intra-radicular infection.

2 *Correct answer B*

3 *Correct answer A*: Acid-etch retained resin-composite restorations are preferred to amalgam as they minimise leakage, especially where the access cavity is surrounded by enamel.

Alomari *et al.* (2001) showed that glass ionomers reduce the cusp deflection that results from curing of resin composite. (Alomari, Q.D., Reinhardt, J.W. and Boyer, D.B. Effect of liners on cusp deflection and gap formation in composite restorations. *Op. Dent.*, 2001, **26**: 406–41).

4 *Correct answer A*: This technique involves the removal of the canal contents from the coronal end of the canal towards the working length. Gates-Glidden burs are used to flare the opening of the canal and remove the pulp tissue followed by successively smaller files. A reaming action is recommended by Morgan and Montgomery (1984) (Morgan, L.F. and Montgomery, S. An evaluation of the crown-down pressureless technique. *J. Endod.*, 1984, **10**: 491–8). Further information can be obtained from the following two references.

Dastmalchi, N., Kazemi, Z., Hashemi, S., Peters, O.A. and Jafarzadeh, H. Definition and endodontic treatment of dilacerated canals: a survey of Diplomates of the American Board of Endodontics. *J. Contemp. Dent. Pract.*, 2011, **12**: 8–13.

Siqueira, J.F. Jr, Rôças, I.N. and Riche, F.N. and Provenzano J.C. Clinical outcome of the endodontic treatment of teeth with apical periodontitis using an antimicrobial protocol. *Oral Surg. Oral Med. Oral Pathol. Oral Radiol. Endod.*, 2008, **106**: 757–62.

5 *Correct answer A*: The technique uses flexible files with blunt tips which are rotated gently in a clockwise direction to engage the dentine. The dentine is removed by rotating the file in an anti-clockwise direction while still maintaining light apical pressure. Anticurvature filing is a different technique whose aim is to avoid strip perforation of the furcation region of molar teeth by preferential filing towards the outer surface of the root. Circumferential filing aims to instrument the available root dentine by filing around the canal. This technique enlarges the apical region of curved canals to allow the access of hypochlorite irrigant and the more complete removal of necrotic debris. Undesirable changes are produced in the shape of curved canals when K-files or reamers are used in an over-zealous manner, because the instrument attempts to straighten and produces a flaring of the apical canal.

6 *Correct answer A*: Bacteria that are present in the root canal can also be found in the surrounding dentine. However, many studies have shown that complete elimination of bacteria in the apical dentine is not possible (see Dalton, B.C., Ørstavik, D., Philips, C., Pettiette, M. and Trope, M. Bacterial reduction with nickel-titanium rotary instrumentation. *J. Endod.*, 1998, **24**: 763–7). *Enterococcus faecalis* is a gram positive commensal organism that colonises the oral cavity, and has been associated with post-endodontic treatment disease. It has been shown to be resistant to calcium hydroxide, sodium hypochlorite and some antibiotics (see Hancock, H.H. 3rd, Sigurdsson, A., Trope, M. and Moiseiwitsch, J. Bacteria isolated after unsuccessful endodontic treatment in a North American population. *Oral Surg. Oral Med. Oral Pathol. Oral Radiol. Endod.*, 2001, **91**: 579–86).

Similarly eradication of debris from irregularly shaped canals cannot always be guaranteed. The remaining dentine wall thickness, after preparation of the root canal, should not be less than 1 mm at any point. This is because plain film radiographs tend to overestimate the amount of remaining dentine (Souza *et al.*, 2008). If a dentine wall thickness of only 0.25 mm is observed, then it is highly likely that a strip perforation is present in the canal (Souza, E.M., Bretas, R.T., Cenci, M.S., Maia-Filho, E.M. and Bonetti-Filho, I. Periapical radiographs overestimate root canal wall thickness during post space preparation. *Int. Endo. J.*, 2008, **41**: 658–63).

7 *Correct answer A*: Carious tissue and friable filling material needs to be removed while providing access to the root canal. This prevents transportation of this material into the canal during its preparation. In some situations, where location of the access cavity is proving

difficult, much information can be gained from using the root emi-nence as a guide to orientation of a root. Rubber dam can then be positioned once the root canal system is located. An access cavity should be gently tapering towards the canal orifice and does not require sound tooth substance to be removed to provide retention for a temporary restoration. The pulp chamber usually provides sufficient retention for the temporary restoration. The objective of the access cavity preparation is to provide straight line access for files to the apical part of the root canal. Although the crown anatomy provides a useful guide to the position of the root canal, a periapical radiograph is also an essential requirement to estimating the pulp canal space.

In a large postal study of Flemish dentists, it was found that three-quarters (77.3%) of the respondents never used rubber dam during endodontics (see Slaus, G. and Bottenberg, P. A survey of endodontic practice amongst Flemish dentists. *Int. Endod. J.*, 2002, **35**: 759–67). The use of rubber dam in endodontics is considered mandatory practice by all learned societies.

8 *Correct answer D*: Inter-appointment flare-up usually occurs with a frequency of less than 10% (Tsesis, I., Faivishevsky, V., Fuss, Z. and Zukerman, O. Flare-ups after endodontic treatment: a meta-analysis of literature. *J. Endod.*, 2008, **34**: 1177–81). A study by Torabinejad *et al.* (1988) showed that those with chronic disease were not more likely to develop inter-appointment flare-ups, but that flare-ups were more common in females aged over 40 years or who had pre-operative symptoms (see Torabinejad, M., Kettering, J.D., McGraw, J.C., Cummings, R.R., Dwyer, T.G. and Tobias, T.S. Factors associated with endodontic interappointment emergencies of teeth with necrotic pulps. *J. Endod.*, 1988, **14**: 261–6). Studies have shown that antibiotics are used inappropriately in general dental practice for the treatment of irreversible pulpitis and acute apical periodontitis, when local measures should suffice (see Yingling, N.M., Byrne, B.E. and Hartwell, G.R. Antibiotic use by members of the American Association of Endodontists in the year 2000; report of a national survey. *J. Endod.*, 2002, **28**: 396–404).

Endodontic treatment of those patients with diabetes would seem to be as likely to succeed as in the rest of the population (see Marotta, P.S., Fontes, T.V., Armada, L., Lima, K.C., Rôças, I.N. and Siqueira, J.F. Jr. Type 2 diabetes mellitus and the prevalence of apical periodontitis and endodontic treatment in an adult Brazilian population. *J. Endod.*, 2012, **38**: 297–300).

9 *Correct answer A*: Sodium hypochlorite has a broad spectrum of antimicrobial activity and is generally used at a 0.5% to 6% concentration, which is alkaline. This concentration will dissolve necrotic tissue and collagen, reducing the flexural strength of dentine following prolonged contact. Ultrasonic instruments can be used to oscillate freely in the root canal transferring energy to the irrigant solution. This removes debris and disrupts the biofilm through hydrodynamic shear stresses (acoustic streaming).

Other antibacterial methodologies include disinfection with photodynamic therapy or ultraviolet light. Studies have shown that using only mechanical preparation of infected root canals will not sterilise them, even if the latest reciprocating or rotary file systems are used (see Martinho, F.C., Gomes, A.P., Fernandes, A.M. *et al.* Clinical comparison of the effectiveness of single-file reciprocating systems and rotary systems for removal of endotoxins and cultivable bacteria from primarily infected root canals. *J. Endod.*, 2014, **40**: 625–9). Antibacterial irrigants such as sodium hypochlorite are essential.

10 *Correct answer A*: In acute periapical periodontitis, some pulp remnants can remain vital but in general the tooth is usually non vital. In chronic periodontitis the tooth is usually vital as the pulpal tissues are not usually affected. In acute periapical periodontitis, the affected tooth usually has a carious lesion and the tooth is tender to applied pressure. In chronic periodontitis, young people can be affected. The classification of chronic periodontitis (not acute periapical periodontitis) classifies periodontal disease as either localised with less than 30% of sites involved or generalised with more than 30% of sites involved. It is further classified according to severity, i.e. slight (1–2 mm of clinical attachment loss), moderate (3–4 mm of attachment loss) and severe (more than 5 mm of attachment loss).

11 *Correct answer B*: Root surface debridement removes cementum and exposes dentinal tubules, but this is unlikely to cause a pulpitis.

12 *Correct answer A*: In teeth with an open apex and necrotic pulp, continued root development can be induced if infection and necrotic tissue are eliminated by irrigating with 1.5% sodium hypochlorite solution. Calcium hydroxide paste is applied as an interim antimicrobial dressing and the root canal is sealed with temporary cement. At a follow-up appointment about 3 to 4 weeks later, bleeding is induced into the root canal by instrumentation of the apical tissues and blood is allowed to flow to within a few millimetres of the cemento-enamel junction. A collagen membrane is applied over the blood clot and a mineral trioxide aggregate plug is applied to the membrane. The cavity is sealed with a permanent restoration.

13 *Correct answer B*: Saliva does have anti-bacterial and mineralising properties, but these will be ineffective in reversing active caries that is progressing through the dentine. Secondary dentine is produced after the tooth has erupted and has developed fully. It is produced slowly by odontoblasts in response to stimuli such as tooth wear. Primary dentine is the major mineral component surrounding the pulp and lying below the enamel. Mantle dentine is the thin, outermost constituent of the primary dentine which is laid down after stimulation from the inner enamel epithelial cells in odontogenesis.

14 *Correct answer*: When suitable radiographs have been taken and an endodontic procedure is planned, the proposed procedure with its possible adverse effects and any alternative treatments are explained to the patient. The first stage in endodontics is to obtain an access cavity and thereby locate the canal orifices. Any damage to the pulpal floor is avoided, but the roof of the pulp chamber must be removed. Coronal flaring removes the bulk of infected coronal tissue and prevents it from being carried into the apical tissues. Apex locating devices can be used for estimation of the working length. The step-back technique involves a method of apical preparation such that accurate adaptation and filling with gutta percha is enabled. Finally, the access cavity is restored.

15 *Correct answer A*: Pontius *et al.* (2013) found that teeth with perforations at or near the osseous crest had the worst prognosis (Pontius, V., Pontius, O., Braun, A., Frankenberger, R. and

Roggendorf, M.J. Retrospective evaluation of perforation repairs in 6 private practices. *J. Endod.*, 2013, **39**: 1346–58). Access and visibility are usually better in the gingival region; the aim is to seal the perforation, but there is an increased likelihood of bacterial contamination. Lateral perforations in this region can often be treated with crown lengthening or diaphragm post and core restorations.

Root perforations in the mid-root region can often be treated non-surgically by placing mineral trioxide aggregate (MTA) over the perforation. A sterile, resorbable collagen membrane is first introduced through the root perforation to form a barrier that prevents overfilling with MTA. An operating microscope is an essential aid to visualise the perforation (see Biswas, M., Mazumdar, D. and Neyogi, A. Non-surgical perforation repair by mineral trioxide aggregate under dental operating microscope. *J. Conserv. Dent.*, 2011, **14**: 83–5).

16 *Correct answer E*: Rotary nickel-titanium files show little sign of wear prior to their breakage, so this is an unreliable predictive sign. Coronal flaring allows a more direct access of the file to the apical region of the root and therefore prevents file separation. The rotary file is used with a gentle pecking motion and is able to rotate freely in the canal before the dentist moves to the next larger size.

17 *Correct answer B*: Apical lesions, limited to the cancellous bone, are not easily detected in plane film radiography. 3-D imaging, as provided by cone-beam computed tomography, has superior sensitivity in detecting a lesion like this, but is not recommended as the first-line imaging technique of choice because of the high radiation dose.

18 *Correct answer D*: Radiography of the root filled tooth and a careful note of clinical symptoms (such as an absence of pain) are both important in determining the success of endodontic treatment. The European Society of Endodontology has produced guidelines* which indicate that if an apical radiolucency persists longer than 4 years, then disease is usually present. However, where the apical radiolucent lesion has been extensive, then successful healing may cause this to reduce but not heal completely, leaving a fibrous scar.

*Quality guidelines for endodontic treatment: consensus report of the European Society of Endodontology. *Int. Endod. J.*, 2006, **39:** 921–30.

19 *Correct answer A*: K-flex files are diamond or rhomboid shaped in cross-section. They are more flexible than K-files and resist fracture when torque tested. K files are square in cross-section. K-flex and K files are rotated in the canal, whereas a Hedstroem file is used in a filing motion by moving the file in and out of the canal.

A patency file is a small K-file (size no. 10) that is gently pushed 1 mm through the apex. The purpose of this is to remove debris that has collected at the apex and allow preparation of this region. Critics of the technique argue that infected material is pushed through the foramen leading to post-treatment pain. However, in an *in vitro* experiment, contaminated patency files that were in contact with sodium hypochlorite solutions had a much reduced risk of inoculation (see Izu, K.H., Thomas, S.J., Zhang, P., Izu, A.E and Michalek, S. Effectiveness of sodium hypochlorite in preventing inoculation of periapical tissues with contaminated patency files. *J. Endod.*, 2004, **30:** 92–4).

20 *Correct answer B*: Loizeaux and Devos found that 15% of dried mandibles contained retromolar foraminae greater than 0.5 mm in diameter and surrounded by cortical bone (Loizeaux, A.D. and Devos, B.J. Inferior alveolar nerve anomaly. *J. Hawaii Dent. Assoc.*, 1981, **12:** 10–11). It is speculation whether these canals contained branches of the long buccal nerve, or divisions of the inferior alveolar nerve prior to its entry into the mandible. However, Carter and Keen (1971) found direct evidence of nerves entering the retromolar fossa and branches then entering the roots of the 3rd or 1st molar teeth (Carter, R.B. and Keen, E.N. The intramandibular course of the inferior alveolar nerve. *J. Anat.*, 1971, **108(Pt 3):** 433–40). However, they only examined eight cadavers.

21 *Correct answer A*: The Gow-Gates technique has been developed because of failure of conventional block anaesthesia if the needle is placed too inferiorly. The Gow-Gates technique places the needle higher in the pterygo-mandibular space. The angle of trajectory of the needle is parallel to a line joining the angle of the mouth to the tragus of the ear and the point of entry is higher than in the standard technique. The needle is aimed at the neck of the condyle, below the lateral pterygoid muscle insertion (see Figure 7.2). The patient has to keep their mouth open during the injection so that the condyle does not move back into the glenoid fossa and away from the needle.

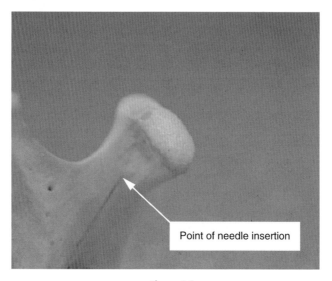

Point of needle insertion

Figure 7.2

22 *Correct answer B*: A fistula is not a contraindication for obturation of the root canal but the tooth should be pain-free. Moisture in the root canal will prevent the root canal sealer from adapting to the root dentine surface. Therefore when the wetness cannot be controlled, the obturation should be postponed. It is not usually possible to eliminate all bacteria from the prepared root canal, but only reduce the numbers to a non-infective level. The reason for this is that the molar root canal is often complex in shape, and circular preparation using rotary instruments will not instrument the complete canal. There areas are often inaccessible to any design of file. In oval canals, both balanced force and circumferential filing do not instrument the whole canal, even when this is performed under ideal laboratory conditions using extracted teeth (see Wu, M.K., van der Sluis, L.W. and Wesselink.

P.R. The capability of two hand instrumentation techniques to remove the inner layer of dentine in oval canals. *Int. Endod. J.*, 2003, **36:** 218–24). The other role of instrumentation is to produce a wide enough canal to allow effective irrigation and placement of a root canal filling.

Internal root resorption generates an irregular resorbed region which is difficult to disinfect, but an intracanal medication such as calcium hydroxide paste will significantly reduce the bacterial numbers. In this situation, a single visit root canal treatment is not ideal. Endosonic irrigation with 1% sodium hypochlorite solution is more effective at removing debris than 0.5% chlorhexidine gluconate (see Cheung, G.S. and Stock, C.J. *In vitro* cleaning ability of root canal irrigants with and without endosonics. *Int. Endod. J.*, 1993, **26:** 334–43). Ultrasonic irrigation (at 25 000 cycles/s) or sonic agitation (at 10 000 cycles/s) involve an agitation of the sodium hypochlorite solution against the walls of the root canal where it removes the biofilm.

23 *Correct answer A*: The anti-inflammatory properties of this material are due to the corticosteroid content (1% triamcinolone). There have been no reports of systemic side effects due to the reduced inflammatory response. Ledermix paste also contains demeclocycline HCl.

24 *Correct answer C*: The effective dose from CBCT is significantly higher than that from conventional radiographic techniques (see Roberts, J.A., Drage, N.A., Davies, J. and Thomas, D.W. Effective dose from cone beam CT examinations in dentistry. *Br. J. Radiol.*, 2009, **82:** 35–40).

25 *Correct answer*: Modern rotary files have multiple progressive tapers along the length of the file, which allow effective cleaning without binding of the whole file against the canal wall. Nickel titanium has the property of super-elasticity and is able to absorb stress during use.

Recent developments in metallurgy have seen marketing of single file systems such as WaveOne (Dentsply Ltd) and Reciproc M (Quality Endodontic Distributors Limited) from M wire. This material has an excellent resistance to cyclic fatigue due to the martensite microstructure which gives it great strength and flexibility (see Alapati, S.B., Brantley, W.A., Iijima, M. *et al.* Metallurgical characterization of a new nickel-titanium wire for rotary endodontic instruments. *J. Endod.*, 2009, **35**: 1589–93). The Endo-Eze AET (Ultradent Products) system is an example of a reciprocating file (i.e. has alternate clockwise and anti-clockwise rotations) that uses M wire.

Protaper Next (Dentsply Ltd) has an asymmetrical rotary action that travels along the file during use. The result is that there is a reduced contact of the file with the canal wall and a reduced possibility of file separation. The file action tends to remove debris coronally. The file is used in an endodontic motor at 300 rpm with a torque setting of 2.8 N/cm.

26 *Correct answer A*: A well-fitting coronal restoration should be placed as soon as possible after root canal treatment is completed.

27 *Correct answer B*: Osteoporosis is characterised by a reduction in bone mineral density in the jaws, but root resorption is not a typical clinical feature.

28 *Correct answer D*: White ProRoot MTA root canal repair material (manufactured by Dentsply Tulsa Dental Specialties) contains bismuth oxide (20%), gypsum (5%) and Portland cement (75%), of which the main constituent is calcium silicate.

29 *Correct answer C*: A periapical radiograph is necessary prior to undertaking endodontic treatment. Obliteration of the pulp chamber is just one of the factors that may complicate endodontic therapy. Others include additional root canals, pulp stones and significant curvature of the root.

30 *Correct answer D*: Teeth which form abutments for bridges should be considered as being of strategic importance. Often, endodontic therapy can be carried out through the crown of the abutment tooth. It is important to assess whether a tooth will be restorable and functional after endodontic treatment.

31 *Correct answer D*: The System B® technique (manufactured by SybronEndo) uses a heating plugger to soften the master gutta percha cone. The cone is then compacted into place using plug-gers. In the Obtura® technique, warm gutta percha is injected into the canal and then compacted into place. Gutta condensers (manufactured by Dentsply) use a reverse action Hedstroem file to thermomechanically compact the gutta percha into position. The main risk associated with the latter technique is that gutta percha is pushed into the periapical region.

32 *Correct answer B*: Peri-radicular surgery may be indicated if a per-foration has occurred that cannot be repaired using conventional orthograde access; it would not be appropriate for the manage-ment of a ledge that had just occurred during instrumentation. Further apical pressure will only increase the depth of the ledge. Both developing ledges and compacted debris will impede the progress of a file in the canal, but it is important to distinguish between the two. Compacted debris is usually removed using irri-gation.

33 *Correct answer A*: Coronal preparation removes a large proportion of the infected pulp contents and allows a working length radio-graph (with a file in position) to be taken subsequently without transporting infected material into the apical canal region.

34 *Correct answer*: This technique prevents the transport of infected material from the coronal canal to the apical region. Coronal flaring using ProFile® orifice shapers (manufactured by Dentsply-Maillefer, Ballaigues, Switzerland) is followed by preparing down the canal using successively smaller files with a watch-winding action. Each file is used to prepare a few millimetres of the canal before moving to a smaller file. When a file has reached to within a few millimetres of the apex, a working length radiograph is taken and apical preparation is then finalised with a no. 25 file.

35 *Correct answer C*: Knowing the expected anatomy of the file canal orifices is often helpful in their location, for example, the dark floor of the pulp chamber is often located at the horizontal posi-tion of the cementoenamel junction. Canal Finders are vertical reciprocating files with a rounded tip to avoid creating a ledge.

They are used to instrument fine canals, after they have been located.

36 *Correct answer*: In this technique, the coronal aspect of the root canal is sealed with a glass ionomer material and the access cavity is left open. The patient applies carbamide peroxide to the access cavity at regular two hour intervals during the day and also to a bleaching tray. The tray is also worn at night. The advantage of this technique is that the bleaching agent gains access to the discoloured tooth both externally and from the access cavity. As a result, the method achieves quick results.

37 *Correct answer A*: The main cause of failure of fibre posts is debonding and the loss of retention (see Rasimick, B.J., Wan, J., Musikant, B.L. and Deutsch, A.S. A review of failure modes in teeth restored with adhesively luted endodontic dowels. *J. Prosthod.*, 2010, **19**: 639–46).

38 *Correct answer D*: Surgical removal of the file is often undertaken when the file separation has taken place in the apical part of a curved canal and direct access is not possible.

39 *Correct answer E*: The tissue around the apical part of the root can be classified histologically as either a cyst or granuloma. Only osteoclasts directly resorb bone.

40 *Correct answer*: A is a called an 'elbow', and B a 'zip'.

CHAPTER 8

Periodontology

Questions

1 Biofilms are a collection of organisms in an extracelleular matrix that grow on a surface. Supragingival plaque is a biofilm mainly composed of
  A gram positive bacteria
  B gram negative bacteria
  C Staphylococci species
  D pathogenic bacteria
  E *Aggregatibacter actinomycetemcomitans*

2 The periodontal tissues comprises
  A the pulp
  B the enamel
  C alveolar bone, root cementum, periodontal ligament and the gingival tissues
  D plaque
  E gustatory epithelium

3 Dental plaque-induced gingivitis
  A is always confined to the gingival tissues
  B can sometimes involve resorption of the alveolar bone
  C may involve resorption of the root cementum
  D may involve the periodontal ligamentary tissues
  E may involve loss of connective tissue attachment of the gingival tissues to the root surface

Review Questions for Dentistry, First Edition. Hugh Devlin.
© 2017 John Wiley & Sons, Ltd. Published 2017 by John Wiley & Sons, Ltd.
Companion Website: www.wiley.com/go/devlin/review_questions_for_dentistry

4 Basic Periodontal Examination is a screening tool for examining the periodontal tissues for bleeding on probing, plaque retentive factors and pocket depth. In this system an asterisk (*) indicates that

A furcation involvement is present

B there is bleeding on probing present

C plaque retentive factors are present

D the pocket depth is greater than 7 mm

E the pocket depth is greater than 3–5 mm

5 If the amount of gingival recession around a tooth is 3 mm and the pocket depth at the same point is 4 mm, the clinical attachment loss is

A 3 mm

B 1 mm

C 7 mm

D 4 mm

E cannot be determined from the information given

6 Systemic antimicrobial therapy with tetracycline is indicated in patients with

A chronic periodontitis and who are pregnant

B chronic periodontal disease as an adjunct to root surface debridement

C chronic periodontitis where they have poor oral hygiene

D impaired hepatic function

E a previous allergic response to doxycline

7 Metronidazole is

A effective against aerobic rather than anaerobic organisms

B used in those patients who are pregnant

C a bacteriostatic drug

D used to treat those with necrotising periodontal disease

E used in adults at a low anti-collagenase dose (20 mg twice a day)

8 Metronidazole can be used as a locally delivered topical gel (Colgate Elyzol 25% dental Gel). With this material

A the same syringe can be used for multiple patients

B one gram of Elyzol gel contains 25 mg of metronidazole

C the gel is usually quickly washed away by saliva

D high therapeutic levels of metronidazole are generally maintained for 24 hours after one application of gel

E can be used routinely instead of conventional periodontal therapy

9 Chlorhexidine mouthwashes

   A have no side effects

   B does not affect bacterial cell permeability or intracellular coagulation of proteins

   C may cause parotid swelling

   D can penetrate into periodontal pockets that are greater than 7 mm in depth

   E contain an anionic compound

10 Root surface debridement

   A is the removal of infected cementum from the root surface

   B tends to cause more discomfort than root planing

   C usually requires local anaesthesia

   D can be used for all teeth in one patient visit

   E fails to disrupt the subgingival biofilm if used with ultrasonic instrumentation

11 Commensal oral bacteria

   A usually cause disease

   B do not usually form part of the plaque flora

   C are usually gram negative, motile and virulent organisms

   D do not usually cause disease and form part of the normal oral microflora

   E are not indigenous organisms

12 Which of the following drugs are risk factors for drug-induced gingival overgrowth?

   A Calcium channel blockers. e.g. nifedipine

   B Aspirin

   C Tacrolimus

   D Anti-hypertensive drug therapy

   E Salbutamol

13 A patient has an isolated 5 mm periodontal pocket around an unrestored lower molar, but the pocket has remained stable for 6 months. No subgingival calculus or bleeding on probing is present. What would be your treatment of choice?

A Subgingival scaling

B Root surface debridement

C Periodontal surgery to investigate for a crack or groove in the root

D Subgingival prophylaxis

E Supra gingival scaling

14 Which of the following is not classified as a 'non plaque-induced gingival disease'?

A Fibrous epulis

B Hereditary gingival fibromatosis

C *Neisseria gonorrhea*-associated lesions

D Lichen planus

E Mucous membrane pemphigoid

15 Which of the following are not considered a significant risk factor in the progression of chronic periodontitis?

A Poorly controlled diabetes mellitus

B Smoking

C Stress

D Many large composite restorations

E The presence of plaque at more than 30% of tooth sites

16 What percentage of affected tooth sites needs to be involved before chronic periodontitis is classified as 'generalised'?

A At least 10%

B At least 15%

C At least 20%

D At least 25%

E At least 30%

17 Severity of chronic periodontitis is measured by the amount of clinical attachment loss around teeth. What amount of clinical attachment loss would constitute 'moderate' periodontal disease?

A Less than 1 mm

B 1–2 mm

C 3–4 mm

D 5 mm

E Greater than 5 mm

18 Classifying the severity of furcation disease on a molar tooth is done by measuring the amount of horizontal clinical attachment loss. What does a 'grade II defect' represent?

A The molar furcation is not involved

B The probe can penetrate more than one-third of the furcal width but does not pass through

C The probe can just penetrate into the defect

D The probe can pass completely through the defect

E The probe can pass 2 mm into the furcal defect

19 A three-walled angular bony defect consists of

A a defect bounded by two remaining bone surfaces and the tooth surface

B a defect bounded by three remaining bone surfaces

C a defect bounded by opposing tooth surfaces and one remaining bone surface

D a defect bounded by one remaining bone surface

E a defect resulting from horizontal bone loss

20 A free gingival graft can be used to treat a localised area of narrow, gingival recession. A free gingival graft consists of

A the epithelial layer, lamina propria and the sub-mucosal layer

B the epithelium layer only

C the epithelium and lamina propria layer

D the lamina propria layer only

E the sub-mucosal layer only

21 Periodontal and periapical lesions can co-exist, which can cause diagnostic errors. Which of the following diagnostic features would be more likely to be associated with a periodontal infection rather than an infection of endodontic origin?

A A history of toothache

B A negative pulp vitality test

C An apical radiolucency

D Vertical bone loss on a periapical radiograph of the tooth

E Loss of apical lamina dura on a periapical radiograph of the tooth

22 Coverage of root recession defects with a connective tissue graft and coronal repositioning of the gingival flap is regarded as the gold standard surgical treatment. Which of the following prognostic factors are likely to influence the outcome?

A The presence of abrasion cavities on the tooth

B The palatal position of the tooth in the arch

C The vitality of the tooth

D The depth of the vestibule

E The level of the interdental periodontal support

23 The prevalence and severity of periodontal diseases in patients infected with human immunodeficiency virus (HIV) have been reduced by the introduction of highly active antiretroviral therapy (HAART). If a patient stops taking the treatment due to drug toxicity

A the HIV will remain undetectable in gingival crevicular fluid

B the HIV infection becomes re-established with measurable viraemia

C the HIV will have been eliminated by HAART

D then this would be considered highly unusual as side effects of these drugs are extremely uncommon

E then subsequent courses of HAART are equally likely to maximally suppress the HIV

24 The biological width is normally about 2 mm in width and consists of the

A epithelial attachment

B epithelial and connective tissue attachments

C connective tissue attachment

D height of the gingival sulcus

E distance from the crown margin to the crest of the alveolar bone

25 The modified Widman flap involves two gingival incisions, labelled A and B in the left diagram below, which allows the removal of a gingival collar. What are these incisions?

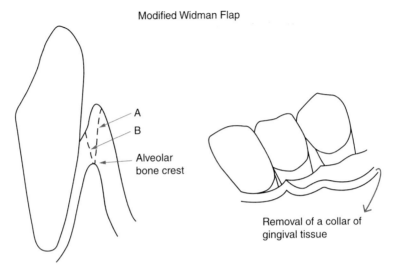

Figure 8.1

26 What are these probes called?

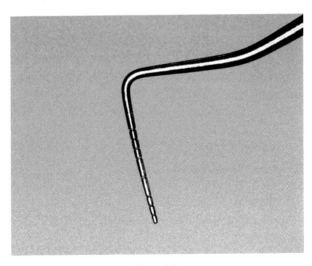

Figure 8.2

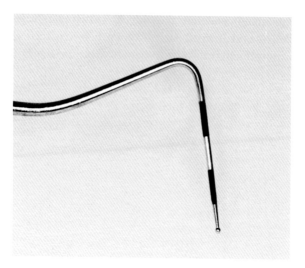

Figure 8.2 *(continued)*

27 Periodontal Diagnosis: Choose the word or phrase from the list of options below, which correctly completes the paragraph.

A junctional epithelium
B connective tissue
C an increased risk
D cemento-enamel junction
E free gingival margin
F 3 mm
G 6 mm
H a decreased risk
I Grade II mobility
J Grade III mobility

Gentle probing usually results in the probe tip being placed in the _____, whereas if the tissues are inflamed the probe tip will be placed in the _____ or even at the alveolar crest. A site which bleeds on repeated occasions with probing of the gingival tissues indicates that it has _____ of active progression of periodontitis. An absence of bleeding on probing indicates that the periodontal tissues have an absence of inflammation. The periodontal attachment loss is calculated as the addition of any gingival recession and the probing pocket depth; the latter measured from the _____. The patient cannot effectively clean probing pocket depths of greater than _____ and they will require active treatment by the dentist. When manipulated with two mirror handles, a tooth which has greater than 1 mm movement horizontally but no apical movement is assigned _____, and _____ mobility if the tooth moves apically.

28 The Basic Periodontal Examination can be used to

A monitor treatment following root surface debridement

B screen all new patients to assess the degree of any subsequent examination

C provide information on loss of attachment in a sextant

D assess the location of furcation involvement within a sextant

E assess whether all the locations affected by periodontitis within the sextant have responded to treatment

29 Localised Aggressive Periodontitis: From the list below, add the missing words which correctly completes the sentence.

A *Aggregatibacter actinomycetemcomitans*

B Leucotoxin

C *Staphylococcus aureus*

D Collagenase

E 250 mg tablets used four times a day for 12–14 days

F 100 mg tablets used once per day for 14 days

G the high prevalence of the disease amongst the general population

H the clustering of the disease amongst family members

I the incisors and first molar teeth

J the premolar and molar teeth

Localised aggressive periodontitis is characterised by the loss of interproximal bone on _____. The subgingival plaque contains large numbers of _____ bacteria. One of the main virulence factors associated with this bacterium is the _____, whose release causes death of white blood cells. This virulent bacterium has been found inside the gingival epithelial cells where it can replicate and then invade adjacent cells. Different strains of these bacteria have been shown to have dissimilar virulence, and the transmission of specific bacterial strains between family members may explain _____. Initial hygiene therapy, involving oral hygiene instruction and calculus and plaque removal, is followed by antibiotic therapy. A typical antibacterial regime uses tetracycline–HCL,

_____ or a locally applied, slow-release tetracycline gel (Dentomycin). Tetracycline should be avoided in children under 12 years and in pregnant women.

30 Choose the cell type from the list below which provides the best fit in the sentences below. Each cell type may be chosen once, more than once or not at all.

a Lymphocytes
b Neutrophils
c Fibroblasts
d Plasma cells
e B lymphocytes
f Osteoclasts
g Pericytes
h Granulation tissue
i Capillaries
j Megakaryocytes
k T lymphocytes
l Macrophages

A The initial gingival lesion is dominated by an infiltration of _____ and _____, which cause the loss of collagen
B The early gingival lesion starts to see the infiltration of
   _____
C The established gingival lesion is characterised by a predominance of _____ and _____. It occurs about two or three weeks after plaque removal measures are stopped
D In the advanced lesion, increased numbers of _____ are present in the gingival connective tissue
E Chronic periodontitis is characterised by alveolar bone loss; bone resorption takes place by the direct action of _____

31 Early detection of periodontal disease can be recognised in children by probing the gingival tissues. What teeth are examined?
A The first permanent molars only
B The central incisors only
C The first permanent molars and upper central incisors
D The first permanent molars and the upper right central incisor and lower left central incisor
E The primary teeth

32 Which of the following graft materials is an example of an autogenous graft material?

A Bone derived from an animal

B Bone from a human donor

C Dense particulate hydroxyapatite

D Bovine anorganic bone

E Bone graft obtained from a site in the same patient

33 In the guided tissue regeneration technique, which cells populate the wound site and differentiate to provide a new periodontal ligament attachment?

A Mucosal epithelial cells

B Endothelial cells

C Cells of the residual periodontal ligament

D Cementoblasts

E Gingival fibroblasts

34 In Papillon-Lefèvre syndrome which of the following is **not** a characteristic clinical presentation?

A Autosomal recessive genetic inheritance

B Severe early onset periodontitis affecting primary and secondary dentitions

C Patient becomes edentulous by early adulthood

D Keratosis of the soles of the feet

E Rampant caries

35 Which of the following statements about primary herpetic gingivostomatitis is incorrect?

A Infection is caused by beta-haemolytic streptococci

B Infection occurs by a virus

C Affected children may feel unwell and have fever and sore throat

D Can be treated in the early stages of the infection with an anti-viral drug (such as acyclovir)

E Is unrelated to plaque accumulation

36 Which of the following statements about the subepithelial connective tissue graft technique is correct?

A In this technique, the recipient site can have periodontal pocketing as this is eliminated by the surgery

B Grafts can be placed over root surface restorations

C The subepithelial connective tissue graft technique can be used successfully where the recession is severe with gross loss of interdental bone

D The graft usually consists of palatal epithelium and connective tissue

E The ideal thickness of the graft is 4 mm

37 In which of the following conditions is gingival enlargement not a typical feature?

A Fibroepithelial polyp

B Pregnancy epulis

C Hereditary gingival fibromatosis

D Giant cell epulis

E Lichen planus

38 Which of the following is unlikely to cause pigmentation of the gingivae or the oral mucosa?

A Peutz-Jeghers syndrome

B Addison's disease

C Minocycline

D Kaposi's sarcoma

E Eosinophilic granuloma

39 Necrotising ulcerative periodontitis (NUP) is characterised by severe gingival recession, ulceration, mobile teeth and alveolar bone loss. Which of the following statements about this condition are incorrect?

A The patient is usually immune-suppressed

B One of the infecting organisms is *Fusobacterium nucleatum*, a normal component of dental plaque

C *Treponema vincentii* is also another important organism in this infection

D NUP has been reported in HIV-infected patients

E Risk factors such as smoking, poor diet, poor nutrition and stress do not play any contributory role in NUP

40 Which of the following statements about the relationship between periodontal disease and diabetes is incorrect?

A In many cross-sectional studies, diabetic patients have an increased prevalence of periodontal disease compared with healthy patients

B In longitudinal studies of children and adults, those with type 1 diabetes have been shown to be more likely to have periodontal attachment loss than healthy patients

C Smoking will exacerbate the risk of periodontal disease in diabetic patients

D Well-controlled diabetic patients with severe periodontal disease should be reviewed annually

E It has been hypothesised that periodontal disease may influence the glycaemic control of diabetes

41 Which of the following statements are incorrect? Gingivectomy can be indicated

A where there is a gingival hypertrophy producing an unattractive appearance

B where there is an intrabony pocket

C in treatment of phenytoin-induced gingival overgrowth

D to regain access to the crown preparation margins following loss of a temporary crown and gingival hypertrophy

E to eliminate a false pocket

42 Which of the following statements about aggressive periodontitis are incorrect?

A The patients are usually elderly with extensive plaque

B Vertical bone defects are present on radiographs

C It usually affects those under 35 years of age

D Often, very little plaque is present

E It affects a small percentage of the population

Answers

1 *Correct answer A*: Supragingival plaque is mainly composed of gram positive bacteria, while subgingival plaque is composed of mainly gram negative organisms, for example *Aggregatibacter actinomycetemcomitans*. With a change in environmental conditions, for example frequent sugar intake, the plaque changes in composition and caries can result. *A. actinomycetemcomitans* is associated with localised aggressive periodontitis. The evidence for this is that this bacterial organism is present in the periodontal lesions in great numbers, produces potent factors that can cause periodontal tissue destruction and produces a strong serum antibody response in the host.

2 *Correct answer C*

3 *Correct answer A*: Gingivitis is defined as an inflammatory disease that is confined to the gingival tissues, whereas periodontal disease leads to loss of connective tissue attachment and alveolar bone loss. Plaque-induced gingivitis may be associated with plaque alone, or may be modified by factors such as systemic factors (e.g. diabetes), medications (e.g. cyclosporin) or malnutrition (e.g. vitamin C deficiency).

4 *Correct answer A*: Guidance from the British Society of Periodontology states that an asterisk indicates furcation involvement irrespective of pocket depth.

5 *Correct answer C*: Attachment loss is the sum of the gingival recession and the pocket depth measured at the same point on the tooth.

6 *Correct answer B*: Doxycline is a tetracycline that can be used at an initial dose of 200 mg, followed by a daily dose of 100 mg, or alternatively in low doses as Periostat (20 mg per taken twice a day). The latter has an anti-collagenase activity. Systemic tetracyclines are contraindicated in those patients with hepatic impairment or who are pregnant or breast feeding. Bacteria in a biofilm are very resistant to antibiotics, so are never used as a substitute for mechanical cleaning (e.g. where the patient has poor oral hygiene and extensive calculus deposits around their

teeth). They may be used in those few sites that do not respond to repeated root surface debridement and where the patient has excellent oral hygiene.

7 *Correct answer D*: Metronidazole is a bacteriocidal drug that is very efficacious in treating necrotising periodontal disease because of its action against anaerobic organisms. It is used in adults at a dose of one 200 mg tablet taken three times daily for 3–7 days.

8 *Correct answer D*: The gel is placed in the periodontal pocket where it becomes gelatinous. It is used as an adjunct where the chronic periodontal lesions have not responded to conventional scaling and root surface debridement. Stoltze (1992) found that the gel was generally at a therapeutic concentration in the pocket 24 hours after single application of the gel (Stoltze, K. Concentration of metronidazole in periodontal pockets after application of a metronidazole 25% dental gel. *Clin. Periodontol.*, 1992, **19(9 Pt 2):** 698–701). One gram of the 25% gel contains 250 mg of metronidazole.

9 *Correct answer C*: Chlorhexidine is a cationic compound that is adsorbed onto tooth and plaque surfaces. However, chlorhexidine cannot penetrate deep periodontal pockets. Patients use chlorhexidine by rinsing twice daily for 30 seconds with 15 mls of solution. It is best for patients to use the solution about 30 minutes after brushing their teeth. Side effects include parotid swelling, tooth staining, altered taste sensation, and desquamative gingivitis. It is often used in the short term by those patients undergoing periodontal surgery and in the long term by those who are physically disabled or wearing orthodontic appliances.

10 *Correct answer D*: Root planing (not root surface debridement) removes cementum and dentine. Root surface debridement disrupts the biofilm using ultrasonic instrumentation. Debridement techniques can be used to treat all the teeth in one visit.

11 *Correct answer D*

12 *Correct answer A*: Tacrolimus is used by the physician as an alternative to ciclosporin in organ transplantation when gingival hypertrophy is problematic.

13 *Correct answer D*

14 *Correct answer A*: The lesions of desquamative gingivitis may occur in mucous membrane pemphigoid, pemphigus vulgaris and lichen planus; they are not classified as plaque-induced diseases. Despite this, elimination of dental plaque and calculus may improve the gingival condition. The fibrous epulis results from chronic irritation from subgingival plaque.

15 *Correct answer D*: After adjusting for age, gender and smoking, several studies have shown an association between financial worries and severe clinical attachment loss (Genco, R.J., Ho, A.W., Kopman, J., Grossi, S.G., Dunford, R.G. and Tedesco, L.A. Models to evaluate the role of stress in periodontal disease. *Ann. Periodontol.*, 1998, **3**: 288–302). Diabetes, smoking and extensive plaque deposits are also significant risk factors for further periodontal bone loss. Any restoration with a ledge or deficient margin will prevent routine plaque removal by the patient, but well contoured restorations do not pose a significant risk in the progression of chronic periodontitis.

16 *Correct answer E*: According to the most recent classification of periodontal disease, at least 30% of tooth sites need to be involved before the disease can be classified as 'generalised'. With affected sites less than 30%, the disease is classified as 'localised' (see 1999 International Workshop for a Classification of Periodontal Diseases and Conditions. Papers. Oak Brook, Illinois, 30 October, 2 November 1999. *Ann. Periodontol.*, 1999, **4i**: 1–112). This is a helpful but an arbitrary threshold figure.

17 *Correct answer C*: 1–2 mm of clinical attachment loss represents mild disease, 3–4 mm is moderate and greater than 5 mm is severe chronic periodontitis. Clinical attachment loss is the summation of the amount of recession and the pocket depth measured with a probe at that point on the tooth.

18 *Correct answer B*: The classification system proposed by Hamp *et al.* (1975) is commonly used (Hamp, S.E., Nyman, S. and Lindhe, J. Periodontal treatment of multirooted teeth. Results after 5 years. *J. Clin. Periodontol.* 1975. **2**: 126–35). With furcation involvement the prognosis of the tooth is reduced because of the increased difficulty of the patient in providing adequate plaque control of the area.

19 *Correct answer B*: The term 'three-walled' bony defect refers to the number of remaining bone surfaces that surround the infrabony defect. Defects can therefore be one-walled, two-walled or three-walled. Horizontal bone loss will not create an infrabony defect.

20 *Correct answer C*

21 *Correct answer D*: A tooth with an infection of periodontal origin is more likely to be vital than a tooth with an endodontic infection. There are studies showing that vertical periodontal bone loss is more prevalent in heavy smokers (see Baljoon. M., Natto, S. and Bergström, J. Long-term effect of smoking on vertical periodontal bone loss. *J. Clin. Periodontol.*, 2005, Jul; **32(7)**: 789–97). Experimental studies on rats have shown that the combination of occlusal trauma and the inhalation of cigarette smoke are both important in causing crestal alveolar bone loss (see Campos, M.L., Corrêa, M.G., Júnior, F.H., Casati, M.Z., Sallum, E.A. and Sallum, A.W. Cigarette smoke inhalation increases the alveolar bone loss caused by primary occlusal trauma in a rat model. *J. Periodont. Res.*, 2014, Apr; **49(2)**: 179–85).

22 *Correct answer E*: Cortellini and Pini Prato (2012) reviewed the literature and found no evidence that abrasion cavities, vitality and position of the teeth or the depth of the vestibule were important prognostic factors in successful coverage of the recession defect. The level of the interdental support and the amount of adjacent keratinised tissue is, however, critical to the success of the surgery (Cortellini, P. and Pini Prato, G. Coronally advanced flap and combination therapy for root coverage. Clinical strategies based on scientific evidence and clinical experience. *Periodontol.*, 2000, 2012, **59**: 158–84). Other factors contributing to a successful outcome include repositioning the flap without any tension in a position 2 mm coronal to the cemento-enamel junction.

23 *Correct answer B:* Antiretroviral therapy is at its most effective when it is given on the first occasion (see Loutfy, M.R. and Walmsley, S.L. Salvage antiretroviral therapy in HIV infection. *Opin. Pharmacother.*, 2002, **3:** 81–90), but unfortunately non-compliance with HAART due to drug toxicity is high (18.4% in study by Yuan *et al.*, 2006 (Yuan, Y., L'italien, G., Mukherjee, J. and Iloeje, U.H. Determinants of discontinuation of initial highly active antiretroviral therapy regimens in a US HIV-infected patient cohort. *HIV Med.*, 2006, **7:** 156–62). The HIV infection is re-established with viraemia.

24 *Correct answer B:* The biological width is the minimum distance required between a crown margin and the alveolar bone crest for periodontal health. A crown margin can be placed in the gingival sulcus for aesthetic reasons, but should not therefore encroach on the junctional epithelium. The ideal position of a crown margin is placement in a supragingival position to avoid risking gingival health.

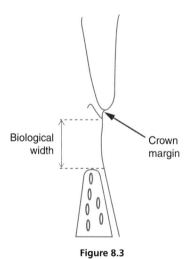

Biological width

Crown margin

Figure 8.3

25 *Correct answer:* A is an internal bevel incision that begins 1 mm from the gingival margin and ends at the alveolar crest.B is a sulcular incision.

26 *Correct answer:* A is a Williams probe (with marked graduations at 1, 2, 3, 5, 7, 8, 9 and 10 mm). It can measure pocket depth.B is a

World Health Organisation Basic Periodontal Examination probe with a ball at the end which is 0.5 mm in diameter. The first black band extends from 3.5 to 5.5 mm.

27 *Correct answer*: Gentle probing usually results in the probe tip being placed in the junctional epithelium, whereas if the tissues are inflamed, the probe tip will be placed in the connective tissue or even at the alveolar crest. A site which bleeds on repeated occasions with probing of the gingival tissues indicates that it has an increased risk of active progression of periodontitis. An absence of bleeding on probing indicates that the periodontal tissues have an absence of inflammation. The periodontal attachment loss is calculated as the addition of any gingival recession and the probing pocket depth, the latter measured from the cemento-enamel junction. The patient cannot effectively clean probing pocket depths of greater than 3 mm and they will require active treatment by the dentist. When manipulated with two mirror handles, a tooth which has greater than 1 mm movement horizontally but no apical movement is assigned grade II mobility, and grade III mobility if the tooth moves apically.

See Corbet E.F. Oral diagnosis and treatment planning: Part 3. Periodontal disease and assessment of risk. *Br. Dent. J.* 2012; **213**: 111–21. doi: 10.1038/sj.bdj.2012.666.

Progression of periodontitis is thought to occur in short bursts of tissue destruction followed by quiescent periods.

28 *Correct answer B*: see http://www.bsperio.org.uk/publications/downloads/39_143748_bpe2011.pdf.

The BPE cannot be used to monitor treatment as it only measures the worst score in a sextant. The disadvantage of the BPE lies in its primary use as a probing pocket depth measurement system; loss of attachment can occur through either gingival recession or true pocket formation. BPE is also unable to distinguish between false and true pockets or provide detailed information about which teeth are affected by furcation involvement within the sextant. Its main use is as a fast and simple system, providing general guidance on the indications for treatment and a suggestion on whether patients should be referred for complex treatment. For young adults (12–17 years of age), it is recommended that the BPE is performed on six index teeth (UR6, UR1, UL6, LL6, LL1 and LR6).

29 *Correct answer*: Localised aggressive periodontitis is characterised by the loss of interproximal bone on the incisors and first molar teeth. The subgingival plaque contains large numbers of *Aggregatibacter actinomycetemcomitans* bacteria. One of the main virulence factors associated with this bacterium is the leucotoxin, whose release causes death of white blood cells. This virulent bacterium has been found inside the gingival epithelial cells where it can replicate and then invade adjacent cells. Different strains of these bacteria have been shown to have dissimilar virulence, and the transmission of specific bacterial strains between family members may explain the clustering of the disease amongst family members. Initial hygiene therapy, involving oral hygiene instruction and calculus and plaque removal, is followed by antibiotic therapy. A typical antibacterial regime uses tetracycline–HCL, 250 mg tablets used four times a day for 12–14 days or a locally applied, slow-release tetracycline gel (Dentomycin). Tetracycline should be avoided in children under 12 years and in pregnant women.

Various systemic antibiotic regimes are recommended for treating localised aggressive periodontitis, involving doxycyline, metronidazole, and combinations of metronidazole and amoxicillin. Management should include oral hygiene instruction and scaling and root planning (with or without flap surgery to gain access to the pocket).

30 *Correct answer*:

  A The initial gingival lesion is dominated by an infiltration of neutrophils and macrophages which cause the loss of collagen

  B The early gingival lesion starts to see the infiltration of T-lymphocytes

  C The established gingival lesion is characterised by a predominance of plasma cells and B-lymphocytes. It occurs about two or three weeks after plaque removal measures are stopped

  D In the advanced lesion, increased numbers of plasma cells are present in the gingival connective tissue

  E Chronic periodontitis is characterised by alveolar bone loss; bone resorption takes place by the direct action of osteoclasts

31 *Correct answer D*: The first permanent molars and the upper right central incisor and lower left central incisor are examined using a modified Basic Periodontal Examination. A score of 4 or * in any quadrant indicates that a full periodontal examination is required. The child may have an aggressive periodontitis, requiring referral to a specialist.

32 *Correct answer E*

33 *Correct answer C*: The cells of the residual periodontal ligament and bone are able to populate the wound and form a new periodontal ligament attachment and cementum on the debrided root. The cells of the mucosal epithelium are excluded by a semi-permeable membrane.

34 *Correct answer E*: Papillon-Lefèvre syndrome results from a genetic mutation that results in the loss of function of cathepsin-C, which is an important enzyme in the intracellular degradation of proteins in inflammatory cells.

35 *Correct answer A*: Primary herpetic gingivostomatitis is caused by a herpes simplex virus and not by streptococcal bacteria. Beta-haemolytic streptococci can cause infection of the gingivae but there are no vesicles formed.

36 *Correct answer D*: The subepithelial connective tissue graft is used in mucogingival surgery. Tissue is transferred usually from the palate to an area of gingival recession. Where the recession is severe with extensive loss of interdental bone, successful coverage of the defect is unlikely. The ideal thickness of the graft is about 2 mm.

37 *Correct answer E*: Lichen planus can affect the gingivae with erosive lesions present (erosive lichen planus), red appearance to the gingivae (desquamative gingivitis) or the gingivae have a white network of striae (reticular pattern). Gingival enlargement is not usually present in lichen planus.

38 *Correct answer E*: The eosinophilic granuloma is the mildest form of the histiocytosis-X group of diseases. Patients may complain of pain, tooth mobility and gingival swelling with delayed healing of a tooth extraction wound and with radiolucency apparent on radiographs.

39 *Correct answer E: Treponema vincentii* is a gram negative, anaerobic organism that can invade the gingival tissues; it has been isolated from the subgingival plaque of shallow periodontal pockets. Smoking, poor oral hygiene, inadequate nutrition and psychological stress are risk factors for NUP. The condition is very painful with rapid destruction of the periodontal tissues.

40 *Correct answer D*: Firatli (1997) showed in a longitudinal study that patients with diabetes had a greater clinical attachment loss than healthy control subjects (Firatli, E. The relationship between clinical periodontal status and insulin-dependent diabetes mellitus. Results after 5 years. *J Periodontol.*, 1997, **68(2):** 136–40). Matthews (2002) recommended that well-controlled diabetic patients with severe periodontal disease should be reviewed every 3 months (with measurement of pocket probing depth, bleeding score and oral hygiene instruction at each visit) (Matthews, D.C. The relationship between diabetes and periodontal disease. *J. Can. Dent. Assoc.*, 2002, **68(3):** 161–4).

41 *Correct answer B*: A false (or pseudo) pocket is defined as one where there is gingival hypertrophy but no bone loss or apical migration of the epithelial attachment. As well as taking phenytoin, ciclosporin (an immunosuppressant) and nifedipine (a calcium channel blocker) can also cause gingival overgrowth.

42 *Correct answer A*

CHAPTER 9

Operative dentistry

Questions

1 Modern high copper amalgams are less susceptible to corrosion than the older low copper alloys because
   A the tin-mercury phase is less susceptible to corrosion
   B the trace elements provide a resistance to corrosion
   C the copper-tin phase is less susceptible to corrosion
   D the increased concentration of silver in the alloy prevents corrosion
   E mercury is partly substituted for gallium

2 In teeth with internal root resorption
   A the tissue apical to the resorbed area is necrotic
   B the resorption starts when all the pulpal tissues have become necrotic
   C the tissue coronal to the resorbed area is not usually inflamed or necrotic
   D the dentine is resorbed by osteoclast-like cells
   E a strong aetiological factor is orthodontic treatment

3 External root resorption is most likely to be caused by
   A acute pulpal inflammation
   B preparing a tooth for a metal-ceramic crown
   C a pulpotomy procedure
   D orthodontic treatment
   E cracked tooth syndrome

Review Questions for Dentistry, First Edition. Hugh Devlin.
© 2017 John Wiley & Sons, Ltd. Published 2017 by John Wiley & Sons, Ltd.
Companion Website: www.wiley.com/go/devlin/review_questions_for_dentistry

4 When reading about the diagnostic ability of methods of assessing the vitality of teeth, you discover that a particular test has a sensitivity of 80%. What does this mean?

   A It means that the test has shown the tooth is definitely vital

   B It means that if you repeated the test 100 times on the same tooth, it would register vitality on 80 occasions

   C It means that the tooth is definitely non-vital

   D It means that if the test was carried out on 100 non-vital teeth, it would register that they were non-vital on 80 occasions

   E It means that if the test was carried out on 100 teeth known to be vital, the test would find 80 of these teeth vital, on average

5 On a bitewing radiograph, a carious lesion is visible on the approximal surface of the upper molar. The tooth needs to be restored if

   A the caries has involved the enamel

   B the caries has not changed in size since a previous radiograph was taken

   C the carious lesion involves the root surface

   D the carious lesion is cavitated and involves the deeper dentine

   E the family relatives have a high caries rate

6 The European guidelines on radiation protection in dental radiology state that when adults are classified as at high risk of caries, they should receive posterior bitewing radiographs

   A at 6-monthly intervals until the individual enters a lower risk category

   B at 9–12 month intervals until the individual enters a lower risk category

   C at 12–18 month intervals until the individual enters a lower risk category

   D at 19–24 month intervals until the individual enters a lower risk category

   E only when caries is present clinically

7 Quantitative laser fluorescence uses incident blue light to illuminate the tooth. The healthy tooth enamel fluoresces a green colour, which is captured by the intra-oral camera, while the blue light is filtered out.

   Quantitative laser fluorescence allows the detection of carious lesions

A which are seen as dark areas over the affected enamel
B because of the decreased scattering of incident light
C but not of hypoplastic lesions
D which are seen as red areas over the affected enamel
E but cannot be used to monitor the enamel remineralisation following regular application of fluoride varnish

8 In a resin composite filling material, the resin component adheres to the inorganic filler by
A covalent bonding
B a vinyl epoxy silane or methyl silane coupling agent
C an inherent bond between the two materials
D hydrogen bonds
E generation of a bond during light exposure

9 Retention of amalgam does not include using
A placement of an undercut box in the dentine
B a bonded amalgam restoration
C dentine pins
D grooves placed into the dentine
E indirect techniques

10 Atraumatic restorative treatment (ART) involves
A removing all the caries from a lesion, including the demineralised dentine
B removing the soft caries with a round bur and restoring with amalgam
C removing all bacteria from the cavity
D removing all soft caries with hand instruments and restoring the cavity with either a glass ionomer or resin-modified glass ionomer restoration
E caries removal that usually requires local anaesthesia

11 Caries-detector dyes, such as 1% acid red in propylene glycol, will
A not stain food debris
B stain the mineralised component of dentine
C not stain the demineralised dentine
D not stain the patient's clothes
E result in over-treatment if used to decide whether to restore operatively a lesion with suspected occlusal caries

12 In carious root surface lesions that have arrested, they usually
  A appear soft when probed
  B have heavily infected dentine
  C appear brown in colour and feel hard when probed
  D lie close to or beneath the gingival margin
  E appear leathery when probed

13 Which cavity liner provides the least post-operative sensitivity beneath amalgam restorations?
  A Cavity varnish
  B Glass ionomer
  C Calcium hydroxide
  D Dentine bonding agent
  E There is no evidence for the superiority of any particular liner

14 The minimum width of an occlusal cavity preparation is limited by the minimum width that can be used in the manufacture of diamond and tungsten carbide burs. The ideal minimum width of a cavity outline is therefore
  A between 0.5 and 0.8 mm
  B between 0.8 and 1 mm
  C between 1 and 1.2 mm
  D between 1.2 and 1.4 mm
  E between 1.4 and 1.5 mm

15 In a class II cavity preparation for amalgam, the occlusal isthmus is kept narrow to allow the opposing dentition to occlude on enamel, where possible. In addition, to maintain the strength of the tooth the occlusal isthmus is
  A prepared to about one-quarter the width of the intercuspal distance
  B prepared to about one-third the width of the intercuspal distance
  C prepared to about one-half the intercuspal distance
  D prepared to between one-quarter and one-third the width of the intercuspal distance
  E prepared to between one-third and one-half the width of the intercuspal distance

16 What is the average life-span of an extensive amalgam restoration placed by an experienced dentist?

A 3–5 years

B 5–8 years

C 10–15 years

D 16–20 years

E Over 20 years

17 What is a three-stage 'total-etch' adhesive system?

A It is a self-etching adhesive system

B A technique where the dentinal smear layer is dissolved by etchant followed by placement of primer and bonding resin

C A technique where the smear layer is removed by an etchant, followed by placement of a hydrophobic primer/resin combination

D It involves a selective etch of enamel, dentine and affected dentine

E It is a system that involves bonding to wet dentine

18 A hydrophilic resin modified glass ionomer (RMGI) undergoes polymerisation shrinkage when cured, but does the hygroscopic expansion subsequently compensate for this?

A The polymerisation shrinkage of RMGI is always less than the hygroscopic expansion

B The polymerisation shrinkage of RMGI is compensated by the hygroscopic expansion within six months

C The polymerisation shrinkage of RMGI is immediately compensated by the hygroscopic expansion

D The polymerisation shrinkage of RMGI is overcompensated by the hygroscopic expansion within a week and can cause tooth cusp deflection

E The polymerisation shrinkage of RMGI is the same as the hygroscopic expansion

19 Abfraction lesions

A result from the propagation of cracks through the cervical enamel

B are caused by toothbrush abrasion

C are shallow, bowl-shaped cervical lesions that affect the molar teeth

    D affect the palatal surfaces of the incisor teeth in patients with bulimia

    E occur at the sites of wear on the occlusal surface

20 During lateral excursion of the mandible to the right side

    A the non-working side condyle rotates

    B there may be a non-working side interference on the right side

    C canine guidance or group function are provided by teeth on the left side

    D the non-working side condyle translates down the articular slope

    E the movement of the mandible is guided by teeth on the non-working side

21 Immediately after placement of a large amalgam restoration in a lower left molar tooth, the amalgam is usually carved so that

    A centric occlusion is coincident with centric relation

    B the teeth meet evenly in centric relation

    C the teeth meet evenly in centric occlusion

    D the amalgam avoids any contact with the opposing tooth

    E all occlusal forces only contact the remaining occlusal enamel

22 Pins are used as an additional method of retaining large amalgam restorations. Which option is correct?

    A Pins can be placed in enamel

    B Pins should be placed in dentine at about 1 mm from the enamel-dentine junction

    C Pins should rarely be placed parallel to the external root surface

    D Pins should engage dentine to a depth of 3–4 mm

    E Pins cannot be adjusted after placement, as this will cause their fracture

23 In 'self-etching' bonding systems

    A etching of the enamel and dentine for 15 seconds is followed by rinsing

    B etching is not followed by rinsing

    C the tooth does not have to be kept free from saliva

    D cavity preparations should have sharp internal line angles to allow easier adaptation of the resin composite

    E the adhesive system contains monomers with a high pH.

24 The treatment of teeth with proximal carious lesions using the 'tunnel technique' and restoration with glass ionomer

A provides good resistance to further demineralisation

B delivers a superior life-span to conventional class II composite and amalgam restorations

C is improved with prior etching of the enamel and dentine with phosphoric acid before restoration placement

D allows effective caries removal

E results in a reduced strength for the marginal ridge

25 A patient returns to consult you as the approximal-occlusal amalgam restoration you placed recently has undergone bulk fracture. What is the most likely factor to have caused this?

A The amalgam was too deep (>1.5 mm in depth)

B The cavo-surface angle was 90°

C Retention grooves were placed in the gingival floor of the cavity preparation

D The internal axio-pulpal line angle was too sharp

E The enamel was undermined

26 In the selective etch technique, what should undergo etching with phosphoric acid?

A the enamel and dentine

B the dentine not overlying the pulp

C the non-friable enamel

D the enamel

E the glass ionomer restoration lining the cavity

27 The International Caries Detection and Assessment System (ICDAS) classifies the clinical presentation of caries in cleaned, dry teeth. A coronal primary carious lesion is suspected and code 3 is used where

A there is some discolouration present following lengthy drying of the tooth

B a carious opacity is present in the enamel

C there is a breakdown of the enamel

D the dentine appears to have a grey shadow under the suspected lesion

E a discrete cavity is present with exposed dentine

28 Caries control. Using the list of options below, choose the best-fitting answer to the questions.

A Daily rinse of 0.05% sodium fluoride and the dentist should apply fluoride varnish 3–4 times per year

B On an annual basis

C The regular inspection appointment (at 3 or 6 month intervals)

D When the permanent teeth start to erupt into the mouth

E Fluoride toothpaste containing 1000 ppm fluoride

F Apply fluoride varnish every 3 months

G Moderate risk of caries

H Severe risk of caries

I High risk of caries

a A young patient aged 12 years is wearing an orthodontic appliance. What preventive agents are used to stop caries developing around the brackets?

b When is the most convenient time to apply fluoride varnish to teeth as part of a caries preventive programme?

c A patient with a dry mouth has developed some early decalcification on the labial surface of the lower incisors. What might the dentist do in preventing the caries developing further?

d In patients that are wearing a fixed orthodontic appliance, in what category of caries risk does this place them, regardless of other factors?

29 At what age is calcification of the maxillary incisors and canines complete?

A 4 years

B 5 years

C 6 years

D 7 years

30 Tooth morphology: The Upper First Molar. From the list of options below, choose the correct answer to complete the sentences in the paragraph.

A 9–10 years

B 7–8 years

C 2.5–3 years

D 6–7 years

E 21–24 months

F the mesiopalatal

G the distopalatal

H the distobuccal

The upper first permanent molar erupts into the mouth when the child is aged _____. The initial calcification of this tooth had begun at around birth, with often a neonatal line present at the cusp tip. Completion of the calcification of the crown occurs at age _____ years. Four major cusps are present on the crown, the largest of which is _____ and the smallest is _____. The roots of the teeth are usually complete by _____. The palatal surface is the most convex of the crown surfaces. This tooth can have more than three root canals.

31 The Lower First Molar: From the list of options below, choose the correct answer to complete the sentences in the paragraph.

A 7 – 8 years

B 6 – 7 years

C 2.5 – 3 years

D 21–24 months

E the mesiobuccal

F the distal

G the mesiolingual

H oblong

I rhomboidal

J oval

The lower first molar erupts into the mouth when the child is aged _____. The initial calcification of this tooth begins at around birth. Completion of the calcification of the crown occurs at age _____. The crown is _____ in shape. Five cusps are present on the crown, usually the _____ is the largest and _____ is the smallest.

32 Which of the following statements is correct?

A Direct pulp capping is when a protective dressing is placed over a small (<1 mm²) pulpal exposure

B Direct pulp capping can still take place if there is continued bleeding

C Direct pulp capping procedures can be used successfully in primary teeth

D The anti-bacterial properties of the dressing used in direct pulp capping will eliminate contamination of the exposed pulp

E Direct pulp capping has a poor success rate

33 Which one of the following statements about dentine hypersensitivity is correct?

A The pain is due to nerves becoming exposed on the dentine surface

B Dentine hypersensitivity does not result from a routine scale and polish

C Treatments using potassium-containing toothpastes have been shown to lack subjective benefit when assessed

D Management may involve tubular exposure and nerve desensitisation

E Patients with toothwear are not at increased risk of dentine hypersensitivity

34 Configuration factor (C-factor) is the ratio of bonded surface to unbonded surface in a cavity preparation for a resin composite restoration. It is important because a high C-factor cavity will have high polymerisation stresses on the adjacent tooth structure during curing of the resin composite. Which of the following cavity designs will have the highest C-factor?

A Class IV cavity

B Class II cavity in a premolar tooth

C A narrow Class I cavity in a molar tooth

D Class II cavity in a molar tooth

E A wide Class I cavity in a molar tooth

35 Which statement is correct?

A Laboratory-processed composite restorations wear more than ceramics

B Laboratory-processed composites wear more than direct composites

C Ceramics wear more than direct composites

D There is no clinically important difference in the wear between enamel, direct composites, ceramics and laboratory-processed composites

36 According to a 2009 Cochrane review, bonding amalgam with an adhesive resin

A is highly cost-effective

B significantly improved the marginal adaptation

C significantly improved the post-operative sensitivity

D improved the fracture resistance of the teeth

E has insufficient evidence of improved retention over 2 years

37 The terminal hinge movement of the mandible involves a rotatory movement around a transverse horizontal axis. About how far does the chin move before the condyle begins to translate down the articulatory eminence?

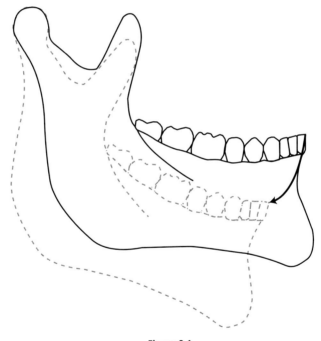

Figure 9.1

38 The health and optimal functioning of the temporomandibular joint is essential to obtaining successful restorations in operative dentistry. In the temporomandibular joint

A the articulatory surface of the joint is covered by hyaline cartilage

B the disc is vascular and innervated in the area in contact with the condyle

C the articulatory disc is attached to the medial and not the lateral pole of the condyle

D the articulatory surface of the joint is covered by fibrocartilage

E the medial pterygoid muscle inserts into the articulatory disc

39 A recent system for treating non-cavitated enamel, interproximal lesions involves infiltrating the caries with resin (Icon®, DMG America, USA). What is used to etch the enamel surface prior to resin infiltration?

A 15% hydrochloric acid

B 37% phosphoric acid

C 17% ethylenediaminetetraacetic acid (EDTA)

D 10.5% citric acid

E 20% phosphoric acid

40 In undertaking the restoration of a cavity with a resin composite, how long is the 37% phosphoric acid gel usually left on the enamel prior to application of a self-etching primer?

A 5 seconds

B 7 seconds

C 15 seconds

D 30 seconds

E 1 minute

Answers

1 *Correct answer C*: The typical concentration of silver in a low copper alloy is about 68–70%, whereas the concentration of silver in a high copper alloy is typically about 40–70%. The silver content may differ between the two alloy types, but the improved corrosion resistance is due to the formation of the copper-tin phase in the high copper alloys. Corrosion in low copper alloys occurs with the tin-mercury phase.

2 *Correct answer D*: Orthodontic treatment may result in excessive forces being applied to the root surfaces of teeth. This may predispose the affected teeth to external cervical resorption or apical resorption, with the latter causing a shortening of the root.

3 *Correct answer D*: Makedonas *et al.* (2009) found that nearly 2% of patients that had completed either removable or fixed appliance orthodontic therapy had severe external root resorption (Makedonas, D., Odman, A. and Hansen, K. Management of root resorption in a large orthodontic clinic. *Swed. Dent. J.*, 2009, **33**: 173–80).

4 *Correct answer E*: Sensitivity measures the proportion of vital teeth that are correctly identified (the true positive fraction). Specificity measures the proportion of non-vital teeth which are correctly identified as such (true negative fraction). The accuracy of a test measures the proportion of true results in the whole sample.

5 *Correct answer D*: Carious lesions should be treated with fluoride therapy and diet advice wherever possible and only restored where the plaque biofilm cannot be removed by the patient. Plaque cannot be removed from a cavitated lesion. Unfortunately, the dentist cannot be sure that cavitation is present on a bitewing radiograph unless the lesion involves the deeper dentine.

6 *Correct answer A*: See *http://ec.europa.eu/energy/nuclear/radio protection/publication/doc/136_en.pdf

7 *Correct answer A*: Unfortunately, quantitative laser fluorescence (QLF) causes fluorescence of hypoplastic and developmental lesions, bacteria and calculus, but this can be distinguished from caries by a clinical examination of the teeth. Plaque is seen as a red discolouration in the QLF image, whereas caries appears as a dark spot on the enamel surface. Caries results in mineral loss in the enamel, which causes an increase in the scattering of incident light and a decrease in the fluorescence. QLF can be used to monitor the remineralisation of early enamel lesions, following preventative and fluoride treatments (Gomez, J., Pretty, I.A., Santarpia, R.P 3rd. *et al.* Quantitative light-induced fluorescence to measure enamel remineralization *in vitro*. *Caries Res.*, 2014, **48:** 223–7).

8 *Correct answer B*: Silane coupling agents are used to adhere the resin matrix to the inorganic filler.

9 *Correct answer E*: Indirect techniques involve fabricating the restoration outside the mouth, whereas amalgam is always placed directly. The alternative answers involve methods of obtaining amalgam retention. Preparing a molar tooth for a Nayyar core involves removing 3–4 mm of gutta percha from the coronal aspect of the root canals using a relatively large Gates Glidden bur (size 4+). Amalgam is condensed into the root canals. These extensions of amalgam provide retention for the core, but they are weak soon after placement and care must be exercised when removing the matrix band so that they are not fractured. Spherical, high copper amalgam alloys have a good early strength and are therefore well suited to this application.

The technique was described in Nayyar, A., Walton, R.E. and Leonard, L.A. An amalgam coronal-radicular dowel and core technique for endodontically treated posterior teeth. *J. Prosthet. Dent.*, 1980, **43:** 511–5. A bonded amalgam technique has since been advocated to reduce the microleakage around the amalgam restorations in molar teeth that have been endodontically treated. An *in vitro* study has shown that this may be effective in the short term (see Howdle, M.D., Fox, K. and Youngson, C.C. An *in vitro* study of coronal microleakage around bonded amalgam coronal-radicular cores in endodontically treated molar teeth. *Quintessence Int.*, 2002, **33:** 22–9). However, no long-term clinical trials of the technique have been published.

10 *Correct answer D*: Atraumatic Restorative treatment does not usually require local anaesthesia, as only soft caries is removed with hand instruments. The technique finds application in those scenarios where the traditional dental technology of the dental clinic is just not available.

11 *Correct answer E*: Early caries in fissures of posterior teeth begins in enamel defects close to the enamel-dentine junction. Caries-detector dyes will tend to stain the early demineralised dentine, resulting in a decision to intervene with operative restorative treatment where this is unnecessary. Diagnosis of occlusal caries should involve visual inspection of the dried, clean tooth, supplemented with bitewing radiography where necessary. Probing the fissure to detect caries is an inaccurate diagnostic method.

12 *Correct answer C*: Carious root surface lesions usually appear brown and feel hard when probed gently. They are usually situated away from the gingival margin and contain little plaque. Root surface caries often occurs in elderly patients with xerostomia. A preventive regime involving improved oral hygiene and high-fluoride containing toothpastes can produce an arrested lesion which is darkly stained and hard. Where necessary, glass ionomer restorations release fluoride slowly and can prevent caries recurrence.

13 *Correct answer E*: There is, at present, inadequate evidence that any particular dental liner provides superior protection against post-operative sensitivity (see Nasser, M. Evidence summary: which dental liners under amalgam restorations are more effective in reducing postoperative sensitivity? *Brit. Dent. J.*, 2011, **210:** 533–7). Liners are usually provided to prevent the ingress of bacteria into the freshly opened dentinal tubules.

14 *Correct answer B*

15 *Correct answer A*: The fracture strength of teeth is progressively reduced with increasing isthmus width (see Dang, N., Meshram, G.K. and Mittal, R.K. Effects of designs of Class 2 preparations on resistance of teeth to fracture. *Indian J. Dent. Res.*, 1997, **8:** 90–4).

16 *Correct answer C:* While some amalgam restorations survive over 20 years, the average survival is about 10–15 years (see Van Nieuwenhuysen, J.P., D'Hoore, W.D., Carvalho, J. and Qvist, V. Long-term evaluation of extensive restorations in permanent teeth. *J. Dent.*, 2003, **31:** 395–405 and Smales, R.J. and Hawthorne, W.S. Long-term survival of extensive amalgams and posterior crowns. *J. Dent.*, 1997, **25:** 225–7). Large amalgam restorations are very durable and tend to survive longer than large resin composite restorations.

17 *Correct answer B:* A three-stage total-etch system involves the sequential placement of etchant, hydrophilic primer and a separate hydrophobic bonding resin. This system has produced consistently high bond strengths which remain stable over time. Total etch systems also produce less microleakage than self-etch systems. 'All-in-one' self-etching adhesive systems have been developed, but they are inferior to the multi-step systems for many reasons, for example the high solvent content prevents an adequately thick layer of resin forming.

18 *Correct answer D:* A study by Versluis *et al.* (2011) has shown that the polymerisation of a hydrophilic RMGI is overcompensated for by the subsequent hygroscopic expansion within a week (Versluis, A., Tantbirojn, D., Lee, M.S., Tu, L.S. and DeLong, R. Can hygroscopic expansion compensate polymerization shrinkage? Part I. Deformation of restored teeth. *Dent. Mat.*, 2011, **27:** 126–133). The polymerisation shrinkage and hygroscopic expansion are greater with RMGI than for resin composites.

19 *Correct answer A:* Abfraction lesions are wedge-shaped and occur at the cervical margin of teeth. Occlusal forces are the main aetiological factor in the progression of cracks through the enamel. The vomiting that can often occur in patients with bulimia is more likely to cause erosion of the palatal surfaces of teeth. Small erosive lesions are diagnosed as smooth, bowl-shaped lesions but when the tooth loss becomes severe, any restorations are seen to protrude above the occlusal surface.

20 *Correct answer D:* During lateral excursion, the working side is the side to which the mandible moves, in this case the right side. The movement of the mandible will be guided by the condyle on the non-working side (the left side) and the teeth on the working side. The left condyle translates down the articular slope. The teeth on the right side provide either canine guidance or group function.

21 *Correct answer C*: If the amalgam is not in any occlusal contact, then the opposing tooth may over-erupt to obtain a more stable position. The amalgam is most stable to occlusal loads when the occlusal surface is flat and has been carved to conform to the existing occlusion (i.e. centric occlusion).

22 *Correct answer B*: Pins should be placed to a depth of 2–3 mm in dentine, about 1 mm from the enamel-dentine junction. The external root surface provides an invaluable clue to the angle of insertion of the pin. After placement, the pins may be adjusted to ensure that they do not protrude out of the restoration and are covered by a sufficient bulk of amalgam (about 2 mm).

23 *Correct answer B*: In self-etching bonding systems, the dentine is first demineralised by acidic monomers (low pH) which also infiltrate the dentine. Rounded internal line angles allow the resin composite to be adapted more easily to the cavity.

24 *Correct answer E*: Tunnel restorations are designed to access the proximal caries from the occlusal surface and therefore preserve the marginal ridge. Unfortunately, the marginal ridge is weakened and is associated with an increased risk of fracture. Caries removal is often compromised due to an inability to completely visualise the lesion. In a literature review involving tunnel restorations (Wiegand, T. and Attin, T. Treatment of proximal caries lesions by tunnel restorations. *Dent. Mat.*, 2007, **23**: 1461–7), it was shown that tunnel restorations restored with glass ionomer have a high annual failure rate (7–10%) and do not survive as long as conventional restorations restored with amalgam or resin composite.

Prior etching of the enamel and dentine with phosphoric acid does not improve the adhesion of glass ionomer restorations, as they are unable to infiltrate into the decalcified dentine due to their high molecular weight (see De Munck, J., Van Landuyt, K.,

Peumans, M. *et al*. A critical review of the durability of adhesion to tooth tissue: methods and results. *J. Dent. Res.*, 2005, **84**: 118–32).

25 *Correct answer D*: Undermined enamel predisposes to tooth fracture and marginal breakdown, but not bulk fracture of the amalgam. Amalgam is a brittle restoration material and sharp internal line angles provide concentration of stress, usually in the isthmus of the restoration. If the restoration is shallow (<1.0 mm thick) then the amalgam may become fractured during mastication. This can be caused by inadvertently inserting thick base materials prior to amalgam placement.

    The ideal cavo-surface angle for an amalgam restoration is 90°. Liners, even under large amalgam restorations, should not exceed 0.5 mm in depth. Where the pulp has been exposed to the oral environment, or nearly so, then placement of a calcium hydroxide with an additional glass ionomer liner seals the exposed area. A dentine bridge is formed beneath the lining. Other direct pulp capping materials, such as mineral trioxide aggregate, have been shown to be successful, but its long setting time is a disadvantage.

26 *Correct answer D*: The selective etch technique refers to etching of enamel with phosphoric acid for 15 seconds, washing off the gel thoroughly and then applying a self-etching primer and adhesive.

27 *Correct answer C*

    Using the ICDAS coding system (freely available at https://www.icdas.org/uploads/ICDAS%20Criteria%20Manual%20Revised%202009_2.pdf), the different options given can be coded as follows:

A There is some discolouration present following lengthy drying of the tooth. CODE 1

B A carious opacity is present in the enamel. CODE 2

C There is a breakdown of the enamel. CODE 3

D The dentine appears to have a grey shadow under the suspected lesion. CODE 4

E A discrete cavity is present with exposed dentine. CODE 5

    The ICDAS system has been further expanded to include restorations and caries diagnosis using a two digit coding system. So, for example, a tooth with a resin composite restoration

(Code 3) and which had a cavity where the dentine was clearly visible (Code 4) would be given the two-digit Code 34. The restoration forms the first digit of the pair and the caries code the second. The important distinction is whether cavitation has taken place or not, as cavity formation usually involves some restorative procedure (unless the cavity is self-cleansing and unlikely to progress). A Code 2 in the caries diagnosis usually involves a carious opacity at the entrance to the fissure, but there is no cavitation. Codes 3 and above involve cavitation with variable extents of the dentine visible at the base of the cavity.

28 **a** *Correct answer A*
   b *Correct answer C*
   c *Correct answer F*
   d *Correct answer G*
   The dentist needs to clean and dry the teeth when inspecting them for carious lesions and after this a small quantity of fluoride varnish can be quickly applied to the teeth. Use less than 0.5 ml in the mixed dentition.

29 *Correct answer D*: This has important clinical implications when prescribing fluoride supplementation so that fluorosis of the front teeth is prevented. For those children aged at least 8 years of age and with active caries, a daily fluoride mouthwash is recommended. Children younger than this may tend to swallow the mouthwash with the possibility that fluorosis results.

30 *Correct answer*: The upper first permanent molar erupts into the mouth when the child is aged 6–7 years. The initial calcification of this tooth had begun at around birth, with often a neonatal line present at the cusp tip. Completion of the calcification of the crown occurs at age 2.5–3 years. Four major cusps are present on the crown, the largest of which is the mesiopalatal and the smallest is the distobuccal. The roots of the teeth are usually complete by 9–10 years. The palatal surface is the most convex of the crown surfaces. This tooth can have more than three root canals.

31 *Correct answer*: The lower first molar erupts into the mouth when the child is aged 6–7 years. The initial calcification of this tooth begins at around birth. Completion of the calcification of the crown occurs at age 2.5–3 years. The crown is oblong in shape. Five cusps are present on the crown, usually the mesiobuccal is the largest and the distal is the smallest.

32 *Correct answer A*: When pulp capping procedures are used in primary teeth there is an accelerated root resorption, resulting in a poor prognosis. In permanent teeth, contamination of the exposed pulp from salivary bacteria or carious dentine considerably reduces the prognosis for direct pulp capping. A direct pulp capping procedure is contraindicated if the patient complained of pre-operative hypersensitivity, the tooth was non-vital or there were radiographic signs of periapical inflammation. With the correct case selection, direct pulp capping is a successful technique. Bogen *et al.* (2008) achieved a 98% success rate in 49 directly pulp capped teeth followed for nine years (Bogen, G., Kim, J.S. and Bakland, L.K. Direct pulp capping with mineral trioxide aggregate: an observational study. *J. Am. Dent. Assoc.*, 2008, **139:** 305–15).

The recommended technique for pulp capping involves placing rubber dam when a small exposure of the pulp seems likely. The carious dentine is removed carefully from around the potential exposure site and then lastly over the exposure site itself. The exposure is irrigated with 3% sodium hypochlorite and sterile water to remove any contamination and then dried. A dressing such as a biosilicate, calcium hydroxide, bioaggregate or mineral trioxide aggregate (MTA) can be used to cover the exposed pulp and the tooth dressed with a resin modified glass ionomer. Self-etching adhesives should not be used as a direct pulp capping material, as they are toxic to the pulp. A hermetic seal is provided with a bonded resin composite restoration and the tooth is reviewed within six months. At the review appointment the patient is asked if they have had any symptoms or discomfort from the tooth, the tooth colour and vitality is checked and the surrounding tissues are examined for a sinus tract or swelling.

33 *Correct answer C*: The cause of dentine hypersensitivity is thought to be due to fluid movement in the dentinal tubules when the surface dentine is exposed to a stimulus. Scaling may cause gingival recession and dentine hypersensitivity. Poulsen *et al.* (2006) in a Cochrane review showed that trials testing the efficacy of potassium containing toothpastes had been performed on small numbers of subjects and the results depended on the methods used to test the treatments (Poulsen, S., Errboe, M., Lescay Mevil, Y. and Glenny, A.M. Potassium-containing toothpastes for dentine hypersensitivity. *Cochrane Database of Systematic Reviews* 2006, **Issue 3**: Art. No.: CD001476. DOI: 10.1002/14651858.CD001476.pub2). Nerve desensitisation and tubular occlusion (not exposure!) are treatment goals.

34 *Correct answer C*: In a class I cavity, the C-factor increases in deeper cavities, whereas as the cavity design gets wider the C-factor is reduced. However, curing an increased volume of resin composite will tend to increase the interfacial stresses.

35 *Correct answer A*

36 *Correct answer E*: The Cochrane review stated that there was insufficient evidence for improved retention following bonding with an adhesive resin (see Fedorowicz, Z., Nasser, M. and Wilson. N. Adhesively-bonded versus non-bonded amalgam restorations for dental caries. *Cochrane Database of Systematic Reviews* 2009, **Issue 4**: Art. No.: CD007517. DOI: 10.1002/14651858.CD007517.pub2).

37 *Correct answer*: The rotation of the condyles is limited to about 12–25 mm before the second stage of opening where the condyle starts to translate as well as undergo further rotation.

38 *Correct answer D*: The superior and inferior heads of the lateral pterygoid fuse into a tendon which inserts into the anteromedial surface of the condylar neck. The superior fibres of the tendon (not the medial pterygoid) insert into the capsule and disc.

39 *Correct answer A*: Paris *et al.* (2007) showed that 15% hydrochloric acid is more effective than 37% phosphoric acid at removing the surface layer to allow subsequent resin penetration. The hydrochloric acid is applied to the tooth for 2 minutes (Paris, S., Meyer-Lueckel, H. and Kielbassam A.M. Resin infiltration of natural caries lesions. *J. Dent. Res.*, 2007, **86**: 662–6).

40 *Correct answer C*: (see Tori, Y., Itou, K., Nishitani, Y,. Ishikawa, S., and Suzuki, K. Effect of phosphoric acid etching prior to self-etching primer application on adhesion of resin composite to enamel and dentine. *Am J Dent.*, 2002, **15**: 305–8.)

CHAPTER 10

Prosthodontics

Questions

1 Tooth tissue loss. From the list of options below, choose the most likely answer to the following questions. Each option may be used once, more than once or not at all.

A Wear caused by contact with the opposing porcelain surfaces of the upper incisor crowns

B Grinding of the lower teeth by the dentist when fitting the provisional restorations for the upper crown

C Excessive consumption of acidified drinks

D Regular use of photographs, study models and indices

E Replacement upper crowns with the palatal surfaces incorporating metal, and designed to incorporate an acceptable anterior guidance. Metal palatal surfaces are less abrasive

F The tooth wear is 'physiological' and therefore normal

G Referral to the patient's physician for any relevant aetiological medical factors, e.g. investigation of acid reflux

H Use of a stabilisation splint

I Fluoride varnish applied to the lower incisors every 4 months

Questions:

a A patient presents with non-carious tooth surface loss with wear limited to the incisal edges of the lower incisors and canines. The dentine is exposed. What is the most likely cause?

b How might non-carious tooth surface loss in general be monitored?

Review Questions for Dentistry, First Edition. Hugh Devlin.
© 2017 John Wiley & Sons, Ltd. Published 2017 by John Wiley & Sons, Ltd.
Companion Website: www.wiley.com/go/devlin/review_questions_for_dentistry

c What should the definitive treatment for the lower incisal tooth wear involve?

d If the patient was a bruxist, what additional preventive measure could be used to prevent further wear?

2 Post Crowns. From the list of options below, choose the most likely answer to the following questions. Each option may be used once, more than once or not at all.

A Cast gold post

B Parallel-sided post

C Threaded parallel-sided post

D Glass fibre-resin post

E A ferrule incorporated within the core

F A glass ionomer core

G An amalgam core

Questions:

a What choice of post-crown system would you make if the post hole was wide and tapered in cross-section? The patient requests the minimum of tooth preparation.

b What is the most retentive post-core system?

c What post system would be preferred to retain a ceramic crown?

d In a lower incisor requiring a post and core, what might be used to increase its fracture resistance and which would also prevent displacement of the post?

3 A refractory (or investment) cast is designed

A to resist low temperatures

B to resist saccharification

C to resist hydrolysis

D to resist high temperatures

E to resist being dissolved by water

4 Peri-implant Disease. From the list of options below, choose the most likely answer in the following statements. Each option may be used once, more than once or not at all.

A an inflammation of the mucosa surrounding an implant

B attachment loss greater than 4 mm

C plaque biofilm

D an air-powder-abrasive system

  E granulation tissue
  F stainless steel scalers
  G a bone substitute and membrane
  H subepithelial connective tissue graft
   I demineralised freeze-dried bone
  J Autogenous bone
      Peri-implant mucositis is defined as_____.
There is no bone loss surrounding the implant, but the condition is common amongst patients with implants. It is treated
non-surgically by mechanical removal of _____,
but avoiding damage to the implant, for example using
_____. Treatment of severe peri-implantitis often
involves a surgical approach with elimination of posterior
implant pockets. In the treatment of peri-implantitis, guided bone
regeneration techniques have been reported as having mixed
success; they involve decontamination of the implant surface and
placement of _____. A typical bone allograft is
_____.

5 Use the most appropriate phrase from the list below to complete
  the sentences in the paragraph below.
  A optimum fit of the crown
  B possible casting errors in the first impression
  C is less than the ideal amount of residual coronal dentine thick-
    ness
  D is no ferrule present on the residual coronal dentine
  E 7 mm
  F 4 mm
  G 2 mm
  H they can be more easily retrieved than cast metal posts
   I strengthen the tooth root
  J the crown
    Two impressions will be needed when restoring an anterior
  tooth with a cast post-core and crown; one for the cast post and
  when this is cemented in place a further impression is taken for
  the crown construction. This provides for _____. Cast
  post and cores are stiffer than fibre posts and are therefore used
  when there _____. These posts are of limited
  use in the molar region due to the curvature of the roots. They
  should therefore only extend up to about _____ into the root

canals. A cast post in an anterior tooth should be at least as long as _____. Fibre posts have the major advantage that _____.

Nayyar amalgam cores are used in posterior teeth. _____ of gutta percha is removed from the root canal orifice to provide retention for the condensed amalgam. This may not be necessary if there is at least _____ of pulpal axial wall present to retain the amalgam.

6 Failure of Ceramic Crowns. Choose the word or phrase from the list of options below which correctly completes the paragraph.
 A compressive
 B tensile
 C leucite-reinforced ceramic
 D lithium disilicate
 E hydrogen fluoride solution
 F solution of 37% phosphoric acid
 G less than 3 mm
 H less than 5 mm
 I a dual-cured resin cement
 J a tribochemical silica coating

Anterior ceramic crowns are fractured when they undergo twisting or _____ forces, as they are brittle materials. These forces cause surface flaws to propagate through the ceramic. Stronger materials with moderate flexural strength such as IPS Empress ® (Ivoclar Vivodent) are composed of a _____. These materials have improved properties due to the compressive forces which develop around the crystals as they cool. These forces tend to deflect cracks. IPS e.max ® (Ivoclar Vivadent) has a high flexural strength and contains _____ crystals. Both of these silica-based ceramic materials can be adhesively bonded to tooth structure by etching the fitting surface with a _____ and applying a silane agent. The restorations are then bonded to the tooth with _____. Lithium disilicate-based ceramic restorations can be used when the tooth has a short clinical crown height of _____ or is over-tapered.

7 In preparing a lightly stained, maxillary central incisor tooth for a veneer restoration that does not cover the incisal edge, the preparation of the labial surface of the tooth involves

A a 0.3 mm reduction over the whole labial surface

B about a 0.5 mm reduction at the mid-labial region and less than 0.3 mm at the gingival margin

C a 0.7 mm reduction over the whole labial surface

D a 0.3 mm reduction at the mid-labial region and 0.5 mm reduction at the gingival margin

E a 1.0 mm reduction over the whole labial surface

8 Metal-Ceramic crown preparation for an upper premolar tooth

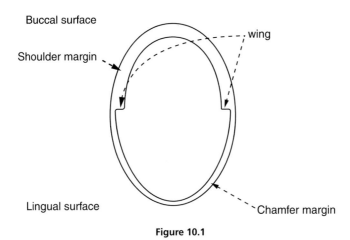

Buccal surface

wing

Shoulder margin

Lingual surface

Chamfer margin

Figure 10.1

Indicate the ideal width of the buccal shoulder preparation for a porcelain-fused-to-metal crown.

A 0.50–0.7 mm

B 0.75–0.95 mm

C 1.00–1.25 mm

D 1.25–1.45 mm

E 1.50 mm

9 The choice of articulator. Choose the articulator type, from the list below, which is the most appropriate to use in the clinical situation described.

A Hinge articulator

B Average value articulator

C Average value articulator with facebow mounting of casts

D Semi-adjustable articulator with facebow mounting of casts

E Fully adjustable articulator

Questions:

a An upper central incisor tooth needs to be prepared for a metal-ceramic crown. The adjacent teeth provide anterior guidance

b All of the upper anterior teeth are to be prepared for metal ceramic crowns, but conforming to the existing occlusion

c The dentist wishes to perform a diagnostic wax-up on selected anterior teeth, but wishes to maintain the patient's existing occlusion (conformative approach)

d A weakened lingual cusp on an over-erupted lower left first molar requires reduction to prevent fracture in the future. Diagnostic casts need to be mounted

10 Preparation of teeth for Metal-Ceramic crowns.

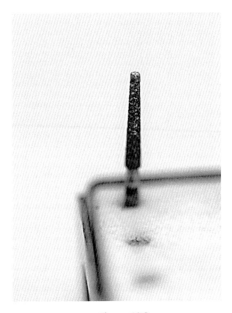

Figure 10.2

This bur is used for preparing the buccal or labial shoulder of metal-ceramic crown preparations. The flat end is 1 mm in diameter and the bur is 10 mm long. At its widest end the bur is 1.5 mm in diameter. What approximate axial taper does this provide for the prepared surface?

A about 1.5°

B 5°

C 7°

D 10°

E 12°

11 In preparing a molar tooth for a metal-ceramic crown with occlusal metal, what is the accepted reduction of height on the functional cusp?

A 0.75 mm

B 1.0 mm

C 1.5 mm

D 2.0 mm

E 2.5 mm

12 What is the ideal margin preparation for a full veneer gold crown?

A Shoulder

B Chamfer

C Bevelled shoulder

D Knife edge margin

E No preparation is needed

13 A patient returns complaining that the gingival tissues around a recently fitted crown are swollen and tender. The gingival tissues bleed on probing. There are no plaque deposits or bleeding on probing elsewhere in the patient's mouth. What is the most likely explanation for the inflammation?

A Poor oral hygiene in the area around the newly fitted crown

B Recurrent caries around the crown margin

C The tooth has become non-vital

D Either that the crown encroaches on the biological width or that the margins are placed sub-gingivally

E The crown cement lute has dissolved

14 Functional cusp bevel on a lower molar tooth

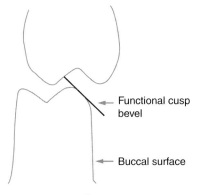

Figure 10.3

The purpose of a functional cusp bevel on a full veneer crown preparation on a lower molar is

A to provide retention to the crown restoration

B to provide an increased inclination of the buccal surface

C to provide the correct contour and thickness of the crown restoration so that working side premature contacts are avoided

D to minimise the amount of tooth reduction needed on the occlusal surface

E to improve the aesthetics of the crown restoration

15 Bleaching of teeth

Choose the word or phrase from the list of options below which correctly completes the paragraph.

A sodium perborate

B teeth with previous trauma

C Sodium fluoride gel

D Externally exposed dentine

E Coronal gutta percha

F Densensitising solution

G Large pulps

H a history of previous dentine sensitivity

I A month

J A week

Bleaching of non-vital teeth involves sealing a bleaching agent such as carbamide peroxide or _____ in the pulp chamber. Root resorption can occur, and the risk is increased in _____ or where heat has been used. The hydrogen peroxide may also increase the potential for dentine to be resorbed. To prevent this, a base of glass ionomer is placed over the _____. With bleaching of vital teeth, those patients _____ may experience increased sensitivity. Placement of acid etched resin composite restorations should be delayed about _____ after bleaching procedures to allow the colour to stabilise and also for the increased oxygen in the enamel to dissipate, as it can inhibit polymerisation.

16 Bonding porcelain veneers to a tooth prepared where all of the enamel has been removed has a high likely of failure because
A the tooth is now more flexible than the porcelain veneer, concentrating the load at the dentine-porcelain bond
B of the occlusal forces with the opposing teeth
C the microleakage between porcelain and dentine will cause loss of retention over time
D of the effect of long-term thermo-cycling changes
E of all of the above

17

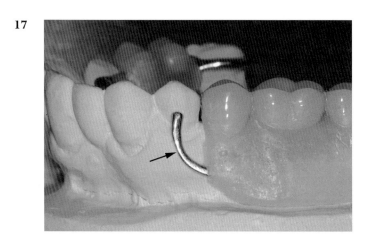

Figure 10.4

In the above photograph, the arrow indicates a gingivally approaching cast cobalt chromium clasp. What is the ideal horizontal depth of undercut engaged by the clasp and what is the minimum clasp length?
A 0.25 mm undercut and 15 mm length
B 0.5 mm undercut and 20 mm length

C 0.25 mm undercut and 7 mm length
D 0.75 mm undercut and 20 mm length
E 0.5 mm undercut and 15 mm length

18 The colour of an all-ceramic restoration
  A is partly determined by the material properties of hue, chroma and value
  B cannot be determined accurately without a spectrophotometer
  C is not influenced by the neighbouring gingival tissues
  D is not influenced by the colour of the underlying tooth structure
  E is not influenced by the thickness and colour of underlying cement

19 What is used to roughen the retentive metal wing of a resin-retained Maryland bridge prior to bonding to the tooth with resin cement?[1]
  A Poly-acrylic acid
  B Phosphoric acid
  C Sandblasting of the surface
  D Hydrofluoric acid
  E Bur preparation

20 What is the name given to this major connector (arrowed)?
  A Lingual plate
  B Split lingual plate
  C Lingual bar
  D Dental connector
  E Kennedy continuous clasp

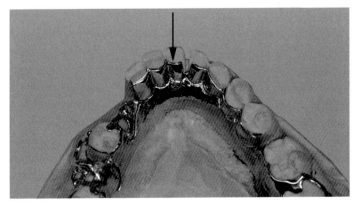

Figure 10.5

21 What is the name given to this major connector (arrowed)?

   A Lingual plate

   B Split lingual plate

   C Lingual bar

   D Dental connector

   E Kennedy continuous clasp

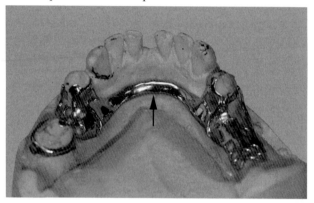

Figure 10.6

22 With all occlusally approaching clasps, the retentive part of the clasp entering the undercut

   A is the terminal two-thirds of the clasp

   B is the terminal quarter of the clasp

   C is the terminal three-quarters of the clasp

   D is the terminal third of the clasp

   E is the terminal half of the clasp

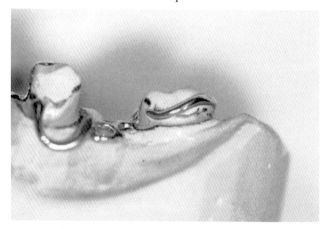

Figure 10.7

23 What is the name given to this type of partial denture? (see Figure 10.8)

   A Hybrid denture

   B Two-part denture

C Sectional denture
D Swing-lock denture
E Precision attachment

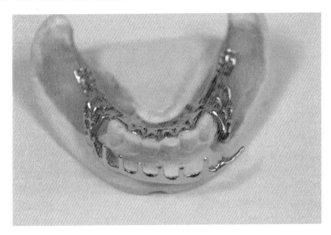

Figure 10.8

24 RPI system
In Figure 10.9 indicate the name and role of the components A, B and C used in the RPI system of partial denture design.

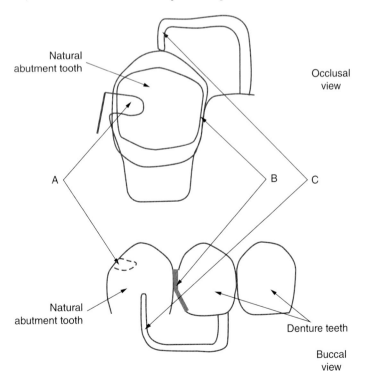

Figure 10.9

25 Design of rests on partial dentures

On a tilted tooth, what are the preferred number of rests or rest design required for optimal loading of the tooth?

A One rest placed on the abutment tooth adjacent to the denture saddle

B Two rests placed on the abutment tooth with one placed adjacent to the saddle and the other on the distal surface of the tooth

C Covering of half of the occlusal surface with an enlarged rest

D Covering of 25% of the occlusal surface with the rest

E The rest is designed to act as an occlusal onlay covering the whole surface

26 Indirect retention is provided by

A the clasps

B the denture saddle

C the lingual bar connector

D the rests

E the sublingual bar connector

27 Which of the following features should be incorporated into an occlusal rest seat preparation on a maxillary premolar tooth?

A 2.5 mm in depth at the marginal ridge

B Flat occlusal floor parallel to the remaining occlusal surface of the tooth

C The outline form of the rests should be circular in shape

D The width of the rest seat at the marginal ridge should be about half that of the intercuspal width

E The rest seat should have sharply defined margins

28 Split-cast mounting is a method of mounting casts on an articulator. The base of the cast is grooved and plaster used to attach it to the mounting plate of the articulator.

The purpose of split-cast mounting is

A to allow verification of the accuracy of the mounting on the articulator, because the casts can be removed and replaced easily

B to facilitate the altered cast technique

C to allow the articulator to correctly duplicate mandibular movements

D to prevent the cast from being detached easily from the mounting plaster

E to be able to distinguish the cast from the mounting plaster

29 Occlusion in complete dentures.

Compensating curves in complete dentures result from the arrangement of the occluding surfaces of the teeth in the medio-lateral and antero-posterior directions. Which statement is correct?

A During lateral excursion, the compensating curve does not reduce the separation of the teeth produced by the condylar guidance

B During lateral excursion, the compensating curve does not reduce the separation of the teeth produced by the incisal guidance

C The compensating curve is identical to the orientation of the occlusal plane

D The antero-posterior compensating curve is made parallel to the ala-tragal line

E Including compensating curves in complete dentures contributes to balanced occlusion

30 Lateral condylar inclination (or Bennett angle)

A This is the angle formed by the movement of the non-working side condyle in the axial plane relative to the sagittal plane

B This is the angle formed by the movement of the working side condyle relative to the sagittal plane

C This angle is formed between the sagittal condylar movements during protrusive and lateral excursions on the non-working side

D Lateral condylar inclination (or Bennett angle) cannot be approximated on an articulator

E Lateral condylar movements are rarely important in planning crown and bridge restorations

31 The 'combination syndrome' may occur when the edentulous maxilla is opposed by mandibular anterior natural teeth. One of the features of this condition is the

A periodontitis involving some of the remaining natural teeth

B resorption and height reduction of the residual ridge overlying the tuberosity region

C over-eruption of the mandibular anterior teeth

D bony undercut in the maxillary anterior labial region

E consistent parallelism of the occlusal plane to the ala-tragal line during complete denture construction

32 The 'BULL' rule is the grinding of the buccal cusp of the upper teeth and the lingual cusp of the lower teeth to obtain balanced occlusion in complete dentures. The BULL rule is used

A to eliminate processing errors after the deflasking of dentures

B to eliminate any premature occlusal contacts on the balancing side

C to eliminate any premature occlusal contacts on the working side

D to eliminate any premature occlusal contacts in protrusion of the mandible

E to eliminate any premature occlusion on the balancing and working side

33 Surveying (Figure 10.10)

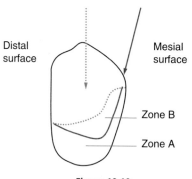

Figure 10.10

This canine has been surveyed in the vertical plane (dotted line) and with a tilted path of insertion (solid line). There are no guides planes present elsewhere on any of the teeth. Both survey lines differ slightly in position on the tooth. The buccal aspect of the tooth is illustrated.

Where should the clasp be placed on the tooth to provide optimal retention?

A Mesial aspect of zone A

B Mid-buccal aspect of zone B

C Mesial aspect of zone B

D Mid-buccal aspect of zone A

E On the distal aspect of the tooth below where the two survey lines meet

34 The Every denture is a mucosa-borne partial denture that has design features whose aim is to prevent lateral displacement forces on the abutment teeth during function. Which design features are incorporated to assist in this aim?

A Guide planes that prevent displacement of the tooth by the clasp

B Maximum palatal coverage of the denture to provide stability

C Balanced occlusion

D Effective reciprocation of the clasps

E Broad contact points between the denture teeth and the natural teeth

35 The impression technique for the altered cast technique

A involves the patient occluding on the partial denture while the impression material sets to avoid disrupting the occlusion

B uses a 2 mm spaced special tray in the free-end saddle area

C requires the patient to make functional movements of their lips during the impression-taking procedure

D aims to apply greater pressure to the mucosal tissues overlying the primary stress-bearing areas of the mandibular free-end saddle

E is most commonly used for the Kennedy class III arch form

36 A complete 'open face' immediate denture

A has a partial labial flange

B has the artificial teeth positioned close to the sockets of the natural anterior tooth predecessors

C is indicated for the replacement of anterior teeth in the lower jaw

D has superior retention to a denture with a flange
E is indicated where either alveoloplasty or alveolectomy procedures are used

37 When processing a set of complete dentures in heat cure acrylic,
   the technician noticed that the two halves of each flask were sep-
   arated by a layer of excess resin which was not removed during
   trial closure. What is the most likely effect that this will have on
   the dentures?
   A The freeway space will be increased
   B Flanges will be overextended by about the same thickness as
      the resin excess
   C The freeway space will be reduced
   D The dentures will no longer fit properly
   E The dentures will have developed contraction porosity

38 The bucco-palatal breadth is the horizontal distance on dentate
   casts from the palatal gingivae to the buccal surface of the ridge.
   On edentulous casts, a fibrous band is seen near the crest of the
   ridge and is thought to represent the remnant of the palatal gingiva. This fibrous band is called the palatal gingival vestige. The
   mean value of the bucco-palatal breadth is used as a guide to the
   positioning of the buccal surface of the artificial teeth in complete dentures. What value of the bucco-palatal breadth is used
   in positioning the buccal surfaces of the upper molar teeth?
   A 6 mm
   B 8 mm
   C 10 mm
   D 12 mm
   E 14 mm

39 A piezograph is a record of
   A the retruded jaw relationship
   B the functional movements of the tongue and cheeks and rep-
      resents the optimal denture space where denture displacement
      should be minimal

   C occlusal contacts in the position of maximum intercuspation of the teeth

   D the duration of survival of tooth restorations

   E the movements of the mandibular condyle during opening

40 The anterior guidance, which you have previously established on temporary anterior crowns, has proven satisfactory for the patient. How would you ensure that the anterior guidance was copied in the definitive restorations?

   A Use a facebow recording to mount the upper and the lower casts

   B Use a fully adjustable articulator

   C Record the anterior guidance using a customised incisal guidance table

   D Record the intercuspal position and provide mandibular protrusive records

   E Adjust the definitive restorations at the chairside to provide the correct anterior guidance

41 In partial denture design, guide planes

   A often occur naturally on teeth

   B improve retention by limiting the paths of insertion/removal of the denture

   C are divergent surfaces on teeth

   D cannot be incorporated into crown restorations as they require too much tooth reduction

   E do not improve denture stability

42 For a patient with anterior teeth affected by localised toothwear, a Dahl technique can be used to create space for restorations. Which of these statements is correct?

   A Resin composite is placed on the occlusal surfaces of the posterior teeth to create space anteriorly

   B The posterior teeth are intruded and the anterior teeth erupt into contact

   C The toothwear was caused by abrasion, attrition, erosion, abfraction or a combination of these factors

D Resin composite has a better wear resistance than enamel, so the patient can be reviewed at about 12 months

E When the molar teeth are separated by 2–3 mm, they quickly erupt and occlude after a few weeks

43 Describe how you would obtain a facebow recording from a fully dentate patient.

44 What is the clinical procedure for rebasing a loose full upper denture?

45 What are the indications for using a copy (or replica) denture technique when replacing a set of complete dentures?

46 Extended matching question. For each question, select the one lettered option that most closely answers the question. The lettered options can be used once, more than once, or not at all.

Options:

A Use a film-holding device

B Use stiffer backing to the film

C Ask another person to hold the film

D Use a sensor positioning aid

E Discard the plastic barrier covering the sensor

F Accept that multiple image retakes may be necessary

G Use an extra-oral imaging technique (eg panoramic imaging)

H Ask another person to hold the film while wearing a protective lead apron

A colleague asks for your advice because they are experiencing the following problems with their radiographic images.

a Scenario 1:

The film is often being bent when held in the mouth by the child patient and the image appears distorted. What would you advise they do to overcome this problem?

b Scenario 2:

Some patients are finding the direct digital sensor is bulky and tending to produce a slight tendency to a gagging response. What is your first choice treatment?

47 What is the mechanism of action of ultrasonic devices in removing posts from the root canal?

   A They cause microcracks in the dentine, thereby weakening the dentine

   B They generate heat that locally melts the cement in that region

   C They transfer vibration down the post that causes the cement lute to fail

   D The water spray washes the cement away

   E The tip mechanically excavates the dentine

48 How can the position of the incisive papilla be used as a guide to positioning the upper anterior teeth in complete denture construction?

Answers

1 a *Correct answer A*

   b *Correct answer D*

   c *Correct answer E*

   d *Correct answer H*: A stabilisation splint is a hard acrylic splint that covers all of the upper maxillary teeth. The occlusal surface of the splint is adjusted to provide an ideal occlusion. The splint eliminates premature contacts, transfers occlusal guidance to the anterior teeth and reduces activity in the masticatory musculature (see Al-Ani, Z., Gray, R.J., Davies, S.J., Sloan, P. and Glenny, A.M. Stabilization splint therapy for the treatment of temporomandibular myofascial pain: a systematic review. *J. Dent. Educ.*, 2005, **69**: 1242–50).

2 a *Correct answer A*

   b *Correct answer C*

   c *Correct answer D*

   d *Correct answer E*: A ferrule is a band of metal that envelopes the supragingival tooth tissue. The remaining coronal tooth structure should be at least 2 mm in height and 1 mm in width. A ferrule reduces the load applied to the root by the post and therefore prevents root fracture.

3 *Correct answer D*: Saccharification describes the metabolism of complex carbohydrate and is therefore an incorrect answer.

4 *Correct answer*: Peri-implant mucositis is defined as an inflammation of the mucosa surrounding an implant. There is no bone loss surrounding the implant, but the condition is common amongst patients with implants. It is treated non-surgically by mechanical removal of the plaque biofilm but avoiding damage to the implant, for example using an air-powder-abrasive system. Treatment of severe peri-implantitis often involves a surgical approach with elimination of posterior implant pockets. In the treatment of peri-implantitis, guided bone regeneration techniques have been reported as having mixed success; they involve decontamination of the implant surface and placement of a bone substitute and membrane. A typical bone allograft is demineralised freeze-dried bone.

Assessment of the peri-implant tissues for early onset of disease involves regular monitoring of plaque control, bleeding on probing, probing depth and whether any suppuration is present. Radiographic assessment may also be important. Regular monitoring is especially important in those with a previous history of chronic periodontal disease. The Cumulative Interceptive Supportive Therapy (CIST) programme has been developed as a comprehensive system that has been shown to be successful in treating peri-implantitis: (see Lang, N.P., Berglundh, T., Heitz-Mayfield, L.J., Pjetursson, B.E., Salvi, G.E. and Sanz, M. Consensus statements and recommended clinical procedures regarding implant survival and complications. *Int. J. Oral Maxillofac. Implants*, 2004, **9 Suppl:** 150–4).

If the patient has probing depths of less than 3 mm, but plaque is present with bleeding on probing, then this is treated with oral hygiene instruction and mechanical cleaning of the implant surfaces (protocol A). With probing depths of 4–5 mm, chlorhexidine is used in the form of mouthwashes, gels and irrigations (protocol B). Where the probing depths around the implant are 5 mm or greater and associated with bleeding on probing, systemic antibiotics (such as metronidazole or metronidazole/amoxicillin) are used for 10 days (protocol C). Surgical treatments (protocol D) are recommended when the >5 mm probing depth is associated with bone loss and bleeding on probing. Surgical treatments should be used with oral hygiene instruction, implant surface debridement and antibiotics.

5 *Correct answer:* Two impressions will be needed when restoring an anterior tooth with a cast post-core and crown; one for the cast post and when this is cemented in place a further impression is taken for the crown construction. This provides for optimum fit of the crown. Cast post and cores are stiffer than fibre posts and are therefore used when there is less than the ideal amount of residual coronal dentine thickness. These posts are of limited use in the molar region due to the curvature of the roots. They should therefore only extend up to about 7 mm into the root canals. A cast post in an anterior tooth should be at least as long as the crown. Fibre posts have the major advantage that they can be more easily retrieved than cast metal posts.

Nayyar amalgam cores are used in posterior teeth. 2 mm of gutta percha is removed from the root canal orifice to provide retention for the condensed amalgam. This may not be necessary if there is at least 4 mm of pulpal axial wall present to retain the amalgam.

To gain the maximum length of post, the gutta percha should be removed to within 4 mm of the root apex. Any more than this and the clinician may disturb the apical seal. Posts do not reinforce teeth; their function is to provide retention for a crown. The increased flexibility of fibre posts may reduce the longevity of a crown where that tooth is subjected to high occlusal loads (see Fernandes, A.S. and Dessai, G.S. Factors affecting the fracture resistance of post-core reconstructed teeth: a review. *Int. J. Prosthodont.*, 2001, **14**: 355–63). Periapical radiographs of the tooth are required before constructing a post-retained crown. To avoid inadvertent perforation of the root, the width of the post should not be wider than one-third the total width of the root.

6 *Correct answer*: Anterior ceramic crowns are fractured when they undergo twisting or tensile forces, as they are brittle materials. These forces cause surface flaws to propagate through the ceramic. Stronger materials with moderate flexural strength such as IPS Empress ® (Ivoclar Vivodent) are composed of a leucite-reinforced ceramic. These materials have improved properties due to the compressive forces which develop around the crystals as they cool. These forces tend to deflect cracks. IPS e.max ® (Ivoclar Vivadent) has a high flexural strength and contains lithium disilicate crystals. Both of these silica-based ceramic materials can be adhesively bonded to tooth structure by etching the fitting surface with a hydrogen fluoride solution and applying a silane agent. The restorations are then bonded to the tooth with a dual-cured resin cement. Lithium disilicate-based ceramic restorations can be used when the tooth has a short clinical crown height of less than 3 mm or is over-tapered.

7 *Correct answer B*: If the tooth is more heavily stained, the veneer will have to be thicker to mask the underlying stain. This will involve preparing the labial surface of the tooth to a depth of about 0.5 mm. The enamel is only about 0.3 mm thick at the gingival margin and the tooth preparation depth for the veneer in this region should not be greater than this.

8 *Correct answer C* (see Blair, F.M,. Wassell R.W., and Steele J.G. Crowns and other extracoronal restorations: Preparations for full veneer crowns. *Br. Dent J.* 2002; **192**: 561–4, 567–71.)

9 **a** *Correct answer B*
   b *Correct answer C*
   c *Correct answer C*
   d *Correct answer B*

Many clinicians use the semi-adjustable articulator with the condylar guidance set at an average angle, which then provides low cusp angles on the crown restorations. The average value articulator is able to provide a simpler and equally effective solution in most situations. With a conformative approach, casts of the patient's existing occlusion can often be used with a customized incisal guidance table to provide canine guidance on the new restorations. Facebow recordings are used in these examples to provide a reference to the occlusal plane and prevent restorations being constructed obliquely at a slope to the occlusal plane. When replacing a missing canine with a bridge, planning with facebow mountings is necessary to ensure that lateral loads during working side contacts are not directed on the pontic but spread over other teeth.

10 *Correct answer A*: The ideal range of total occlusal convergence angle (TOC) for crown preparations is 4° to 10° and will be twice the axial taper on each side of the tooth. The TOC is the angle formed between opposing axial walls of a preparation. TOC affects the retention of a preparation, but many studies have shown that dentists and students tend to over-taper their preparations (see Yoon, S.S., Cheong, C., Preisser, J. Jr, Jun, S., Chang, B.M. and Wright, R.F. Measurement of total occlusal convergence of three different tooth preparations in four different planes by dental students. *J. Prosthet. Dent.*, 2014, **pii:** S0022–3913(14)00099–7. doi: 10.1016/j.prosdent.2014.01.021). Even under optimum operative technique laboratory conditions, students achieve mean TOC angles of 15°. A pencil forms an angle of about 20° at the tip, which would be easily recognised as over-tapered if this was a crown preparation. However, dentists regularly achieve this convergence angle when preparing teeth in patients' mouths. When assessing whether undercut is present on a crown preparation, the dentist positions the mirror so that he can observe opposing sides of the tooth. However, the limited space in the patient's mouth often means that the dentist's mirror is placed near to the preparation. This has the consequence that to ensure the opposing walls are convergent, the dentist will tend to over-taper the tooth.

In addition, the separation of the opposing walls increases the difficulty of providing the correct convergence angle. The over-taper of a pencil tip is easily recognised because it converges at a point, whereas the tooth has convergent walls which are separated by the tooth width and the correct taper is much more difficult to visualise. The use of dental magnifying loupes may help to avoid over-taper. The use of real time video magnification has been shown to be helpful in teaching students the correct taper in full veneer crown preparations (see Robinson, P. and Lee, J.W. The use of real time video magnification for the pre-clinical teaching of crown preparations. *Br. Dent. J.*, 2001, **190:** 506–10).

Resistance form is different from retention (which depends on the area of the preparation), as it predicts whether a restoration will be tilted off the tooth during function. An acceptable resistance form or taper of the preparation is dependent on the height of the preparation and the width of the tooth. The maximum acceptable average taper for premolars is 10° and 8.4° for molars (see Parker, M.H., Calverley, M.J., Gardner, F.M. and Gunderson, R.B. New guidelines for preparation taper. *J. Prosthodont.*, 1993, Mar; **2(1):** 61–6).

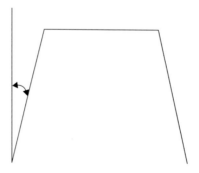

Figure 10.11

The angle illustrated in this figure represents the average taper of a crown restoration. The bur should held in the long axis of the tooth during the tooth preparation to provide the correct convergence angle. Surface reflecting mirrors are useful and the preparation should be viewed with one eye closed.

11 *Correct answer C*: With occlusal metal, the reduction recommended is 1.5 mm, but 2.0 mm if the metal is also veneered with porcelain. This is the traditional reduction that is recommended for good aesthetics, and insufficient reduction will result in a crown that is bulky and overcontoured. Reduction of this width can compromise tooth vitality and strength.

12 *Correct answer B*: Chamfer margin provides the best preparation because it is conservative, provides a readily detectable marginal edge for the technician during construction and a margin which does not distort under load.

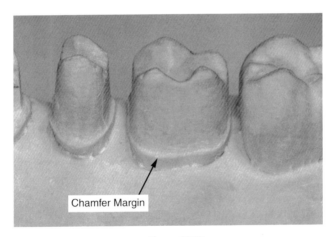

Chamfer Margin

Figure 10.12

13 *Correct answer D*

14 *Correct answer C*: It is important that sufficient thickness is provided for the crown in the region of the functional cusp, an area subject to high occlusal forces. After the functional cusp is reduced, it must be demonstrated not to be in occlusal interference in lateral excursions.

15 *Correct answer*: Bleaching of non-vital teeth involves sealing a bleaching agent such as carbamide peroxide or sodium perborate in the pulp chamber. Root resorption can occur, and the risk is increased in teeth with previous trauma or where heat has been used. The hydrogen peroxide may also increase the potential for dentine to be resorbed. To prevent this, a base of glass ionomer is placed over the coronal gutta percha. With bleaching of vital teeth, those patients with a history of previous dentine sensitivity may experience increased sensitivity. Placement of acid etched resin composite restorations should be delayed for about a week after bleaching procedures to allow the colour to stabilise and also for the increased oxygen in the enamel to dissipate as it can inhibit polymerisation.

Large pulps do not predispose to increased sensitivity following bleaching (see Nathanson, D. and Parra, C. Bleaching vital teeth: a review and clinical study. *Compend. Contin. Educ. Dent.*, 1987, **8**: 490–7). The shade of the bleached teeth may tend to regress to the original shade after varying lengths of time, depending on whether the patient smokes or consumes chromogenic foods.

16 *Correct answer E*

17 *Correct answer A*: If no undercut is present on the tooth, resin composite needs to be applied to the buccal surface of the tooth to create sufficient undercut. If buccal bony tissue undercut is present, the clasp arm has to be positioned away from the tissues so that the denture can be inserted. This can result in the clasp arm being excessively prominent and traumatising the patient's cheek. In addition, a minimum of 4 mm of sulcus depth is needed to accommodate the clasp arm. Clasps that are constructed in wrought wire should be at least 7 mm in length.

A cobalt-chromium clasp engaging a 0.25 mm undercut needs to be at least 15 mm in length to avoid being deformed, and therefore can be used with either premolar or molar teeth.

18 *Correct answer A*: Spectrophotometers have the advantage over visual assessment, in that they provide a more consistent agreement on repeated testing[1], but evidence is divided as to whether they are more accurate. The colour of the gingival tissues and the underlying tooth structure both affect the restoration colour.[2]

1. Derdilopoulou, F.V., Zantner, C., Neumann, K. and Kielbassa, A.M. Evaluation of visual and spectrophotometric shade analyses: a clinical comparison of 3758 teeth. *Int. J. Prosthodont.,* 2007, **20:** 414–6.
2. Wang. J., Lin, J., Seliger, A., Gil, M., da Silva, J.D. and Ishhikawa-Nagai, S. Color effects of gingiva on cervical regions of all-ceramic crowns. *J. Esthet. Restor. Dent.,* 2013, **25:** 254–62.

19 *Correct answer C:* See Burke, F.J. Resin-retained bridges: fibre-reinforced versus metal. *Dent. Update,* 2008, **35:** 521–2, 524–6.

20 *Correct answer B*

21 *Correct answer C*

22 *Correct answer D:* If more than the terminal third of the occlusally approaching clasp enters the undercut then either the clasp may be deformed or the denture will be difficult to remove. The clasp is positioned more than 1 mm from the gingival margin to prevent traumatising the tissue. For an occlusally approaching clasp to engage a 0.25 mm undercut without deforming, it needs to be at least 15 mm in length. This limits the use of this clasp to molar teeth.

23 *Correct answer D*

24 *Correct answer:*
A is a mesial rest providing support for the denture.
B is a distal plate which disengages from the tooth surface during loading of the free-end saddle by moving into the distal undercut.
C is a gingivally approaching I-bar clasp, which engages the buccal surface of the tooth. The clasp engages the most prominent aspect of the tooth surface so that when the saddle is loaded it rotates away from the tooth.

25 *Correct answer B:* There is often insufficient occlusal space to provide an extensive onlay restoration. Two rest seats are usually preferred as they provide a force that is more directed along the long axis of the tooth than a single rest.

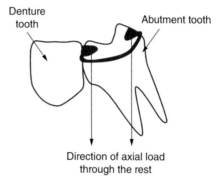

Figure 10.13

26 *Correct answer D*: If a patient bites into a sticky food and then separates their teeth, the denture base is pulled away from the tissues. The clasp will resist this movement and the denture will then tend to rotate around the clasp axis, a line joining the tips of the clasps on opposite sides of the arch. To prevent this rotation a rest or major connector contacting the teeth must be placed on the opposite side of the clasp axis from the displacing saddle. In the diagram, a lingual plate connector provides indirect retention.

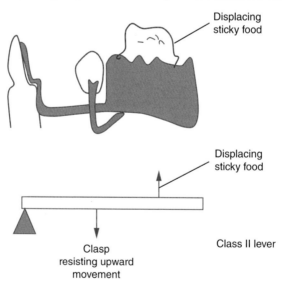

Figure 10.14

27 *Correct answer D*: As described by Culwick *et al.* (2000), the rest seat preparation should be triangular in shape with smooth rather than sharp margins (Culwick, P.F., Howell, P.G., Faigenblum, M.J. The size of occlusal rest seats prepared for removable partial dentures. *Br. Dent. J.*, 2000, **189**: 318–22). The floor of the rest seat preparation should incline gently towards the centre of the tooth. At the marginal ridge a 1–1.5 mm reduction is made for adequate strength of the cast metal rest. If there is insufficient clearance from the opposing cusp then this cusp should be reduced in preference to deepening the rest seat preparation. The maximum rest width at the marginal ridge is about one third the tooth width and about half the intercuspal width.

28 *Correct answer A*

29 *Correct answer E*: The factors influencing balanced articulation are the cusp angles of the posterior teeth, incisal guidance, occlusal plane orientation, condylar guidance and the compensating curves.

30 *Correct answer A*: Fischer's angle is the angle formed between the sagittal condylar movements during protrusive and lateral excursions on the non-working side. The lateral condylar guidance (L) is approximated using the formula: $L = H/8 + 12$, where H is the horizontal condylar guidance. For example, if $H = 30°$ then $L = 15°$. A consideration of lateral condylar inclination is important to consider in constructing crowns to avoid cuspal interferences.

31 *Correct answer C*: There is enlargement of the tuberosity region together with resorption of the anterior labial region. The mandibular teeth tend to over-erupt. Constructing a new complete maxillary denture will involve a compromise in the position of the occlusal plane, and will rarely result in it being parallel to the ala-tragal line.

32 *Correct answer C*: In a normal arrangement of the posterior teeth, the buccal and lingual cusps of the upper and lower dentures are in contact during movement towards the working side. Grinding the buccal cusps of the upper teeth and the lingual cusps of the lower teeth (BULL rule) allows any premature occlusal contacts to be eliminated on the working side and the teeth on the balancing side to come into contact. This preserves the occlusal vertical dimension of the dentures when the patient's jaw returns to the intercuspal position. To obtain balanced occlusion of the teeth during protrusive movements, some grinding of the labial surfaces of the lower anterior teeth may need to be undertaken. After processing, complete dentures can be remounted on the articulator using a wax interocclusal record (to record the retruded jaw relationship) and a facebow recording. Cusps that are premature in both the retruded jaw relationship and in lateral excursive movements of the articulator should be reduced. Where the cusp is premature in the retruded jaw relationship only, the opposing fossa should be reduced.

Occlusal balance is where there is simultaneous contact of the teeth on both sides of the mouth during lateral excursions. It is determined during setting of the teeth for the wax try-in by the incisal guidance, condylar guidance, cusp angle, the plane of occlusion and the compensating curve. Recent reviews have concluded that bilateral balanced articulation in complete dentures is not essential for satisfactory function in the majority of patients (see Carlsson, G.E. Critical review of some dogmas in prosthodontics. *J. Prosthodont. Res.*, 2009, **53**: 3–10). There are also no advantages to using a facebow to mount the upper cast rather than using average settings on the articulator. This considerably simplifies the treatment and reduces costs.

33 *Correct answer*: On the distal aspect of the tooth below where the two survey lines meet.

Placing a clasp in zone A (below where the survey lines meet on the distal surface) will mean that the denture clasp will resist displacement vertically and along the path of insertion. Placing the clasp on the mesial or mid-buccal surfaces of zone A and ignoring the dotted survey line, may mean that the clasp is distorted in vertical insertion if the undercut is too great relative to that survey line. This could occur if the denture is bitten into position by the patient. Without guide planes, the partial denture has to resist displacement vertically and along the path of insertion, therefore a clasp must be optimally positioned with respect to both survey lines.

If guide planes are present that dictate the path of insertion in the direction of the solid line arrow, then the denture can only be inserted and removed in this direction. In this situation the vertical survey line (dotted survey line) can be ignored. The clasp is placed in the optimal undercut of zone A.

34 *Correct answer B*: The Every denture minimises damaging lateral forces on teeth by avoiding clasps. Denture retention is facilitated by frictional contact of the denture and natural teeth. Tooth displacement is reduced by avoiding palatal coverage of the teeth and having wide embrasures and only a limited extent of touching of the denture and natural teeth at the contact point. The occlusion of the denture teeth is arranged so that the teeth are not displaced during lateral excursive movements. Bracing of the denture is provided by wire stabilisers which contact the distal surfaces of the terminal posterior teeth. The other main feature in the design is maximum palatal coverage.

35 *Correct answer D*: The altered cast technique is most commonly used for the mandibular Kennedy class I or II arches. The aim of the technique is to apply a greater load (within physiological limits) to the buccal shelf and residual ridges (i.e. the primary support areas). A baseplate, attached to the metal framework, is used to take an impression of these tissues in the mouth. The casting is seated in the patient's mouth with gentle pressure applied to the metal framework only. The original cast is altered to receive the new impression.

36 *Correct answer B*: In an open face denture, the artificial anterior teeth are positioned close to the sockets of the natural predecessors. An open face denture is therefore contraindicated where either an alveoloplasty or alveolectomy is used. No labial flange is used in an open face denture, which means that retention is often poor. In the lower jaw, open face immediate dentures are especially poorly retentive.

37 *Correct answer C*: The excess resin will have caused an increase in the occlusal vertical dimension of the dentures. The fit and retention of the dentures should remain relatively unaffected. Contraction porosity occurs when shrinkage of the resin occurs during processing, with the formation of voids. This is usually prevented by maintaining pressure on the acrylic dough during processing (e.g. by having excess resin).

38 *Correct answer D*: The buccal surfaces of the upper molar teeth are positioned 12 mm from the palatal gingival vestige and therefore buccal to the crest of the residual ridge.

39 *Correct answer B*: A piezograph results from an edentulous patient moulding a slow setting material in their mouth with functional movements and thereby allowing the neutral zone to be visualised. It is therefore used to record the optimal shape of the lower denture.

40 *Correct answer C*: The anterior guidance, provided with temporary crowns, can be copied on an articulator using the customised incisal guidance technique. This involves first articulating the study casts and then placing acrylic resin over the incisal guidance table. The upper cast is moved laterally from side to side with the anterior teeth in contact, while the incisal pin traces these movements in the acrylic resin. Recording the intercuspal position and protrusive mandibular movements will not allow the anterior guidance to be copied in the definitive restorations.

Using a facebow recording allows the relationship between the condyles and the maxillary teeth to be recorded. The relationship is then transferred to an articulator so that the upper cast is orientated in the same manner to the hinge axis of the articulator.

41 *Correct answer B*

42 *Correct answer C*: The Dahl technique involves placing resin composite on the palatal surfaces of the upper incisor teeth and the incisal edges of the mandibular teeth with the result that the molar teeth are separated by 2–3 mm. The molar teeth re-erupt and usually occlude after 3–6 months. The patient should be reviewed at this time. The restorations may have to be repaired and polished. Enamel has a better wear resistance than resin composite. The advantage of this technique is that it is non-invasive and reversible with the option for more invasive treatments should this prove necessary. For those patients who are unsatisfied with the aesthetic result from the Dahl technique, crown lengthening and all-ceramic crowns are an alternative but more expensive and invasive option.

43 *Correct answer*: Wax is softened in hot water and wrapped around the bite fork. The bite fork is positioned on the upper teeth with the central marking located between the incisor teeth. The handle of the bite fork is attached to the facebow using an adjustable joint, and the anterior locator of the facebow is positioned over an anterior reference point. All of the adjusting screws are tightened. Condylar rods placed either in or close to the external auditory meatus provide the posterior reference point. The condylar rods are loosened and the facebow is removed.

44 *Correct answer*: Denture relines or rebasing techniques should be used when the denture has lost its adaptation to the underlying tissues. The clinical procedure involves assessing the denture to ensure that there are no occlusal premature contacts present. Any undercuts are removed from the denture so that the technician can remove the denture intact from the stone cast. The periphery is adjusted by either removing areas of overextended acrylic or adding green-stick composition to extend the flange. Adhesive is coated over the fitting surface of the denture. A low viscosity silicone impression material is placed in the fitting surface of the denture and then seated in the patient's mouth. Following border moulding procedures to the flange, the patient is asked to close into the retruded contact position until the impression material has set. The denture is removed and the impression is inspected.

45 *Correct answer*: Explanation:
   A To provide a second or 'spare set' of dentures
   B When there has been a loss of fit of the dentures with a mild increase in the freeway space (or interocclusal clearance)
   C Deterioration of the acrylic base, for example bleaching of the acrylic due to the use of inappropriate cleaning methods, but everything else about the denture is satisfactory
   D Where the patient has shown that they cannot adjust to new dentures. Often the new dentures have no obvious design fault but differ markedly from the patient's existing dentures

46 a *Correct answer A*

   b *Correct answer D*: As a first choice, use of a sensor positioning aid will help maintain a secure position and might reduce the slight tendency to a gag reflex. If this fails it may be necessary to resort to an extra-oral imaging technique (i.e. panoramic radiography), but field size limitation should be used if available.

47 *Correct answer C*: Cracking of the dentine and heat production are unfortunate complications of ultrasonic treatment, but are not the mechanism of post removal. Cast custom posts and fibre posts are usually more difficult to remove using this technique. Using post pullers can cause root fracture.

   The Masserann Kit (Micromega, France) is a post removal device which does not generate too much force or excessive heat. The technique involves using a trepan to prepare a narrow gutter around the fractured post for about one-third to half its length. Then the post is gripped by a slightly smaller trepan and gently pulled out with an anti-clockwise motion.

48 *Correct answer*: If the position of the artificial teeth is to copy that of the natural dentition:
1. The line connecting the tips of the upper canines should lie close to the centre of the incisive papilla.
2. The labial surface of the central incisor should be about 10 mm in front of the middle of the incisive papilla (see Isa, Z.M. and Abdulhadi, L.M. Relationship of maxillary incisors in complete dentures to the incisive papilla. *J. Oral Sci.*, 2012, **54(2)**: 159–63).

CHAPTER 11

Medical and surgical aspects of oral and dental health

Questions

1 A patient with a diagnosis of 'temporo-mandibular joint (TMJ) disc displacement with reduction' is most likely to suffer from which one of the following signs or symptoms
   A A history of jaw locking on opening
   B Crepitus
   C An anterior open bite
   D A moderate sclerosis of the articular eminence evident on radiography
   E Clicking observed on either opening or closing the jaw

2 Temporomandibular joint disease. For each of the following patient's symptoms, history and/or clinical observations, select the most likely diagnosis from the list below. Each option may be used once, more than once, or not at all.
   A Disc displacement with reduction
   B Disc displacement without reduction, with limited opening
   C Condylar neck fracture of the right side
   D Osteoarthritis of the temporo-mandibular joint
   E Rheumatoid arthritis affecting the temporo-mandibular joint
   What is the correct diagnosis?

   a A patient has severe pain and clicking, particularly associated with the left temporo-mandibular joint. The joint is tender

Review Questions for Dentistry, First Edition. Hugh Devlin.
© 2017 John Wiley & Sons, Ltd. Published 2017 by John Wiley & Sons, Ltd.
Companion Website: www.wiley.com/go/devlin/review_questions_for_dentistry

to palpation. The clicking occurs when the patient opens and closes his mouth. The occlusion was undisturbed. No trismus was present.

b A patient has pain associated with the left temporo-mandibular joint, with the pain becoming worse during the day. The patient complained of a 'crunching' or 'grating' noise from his joint that had occurred recently.

c There is an abnormal contact of the teeth on the right side only, whereas previously all the teeth were in intercuspal occlusion. The midline of the mandibular teeth has shifted to the right side.

3 Treatment of patients with kidney disease. From the list of options below, select the most likely answer. Each option may be used once, more than once, or not at all.

A Paracetamol

B Non-steroidal anti-inflammatory drugs

C Most appropriate time for routine dental treatment is after the patient has received the renal transplant

D Most appropriate time for routine dental treatment is before the patient has received the renal transplant

E Metabolic acidosis

F Nausea and vomiting

G By way of the renin-angiotensin-aldosterone system

H Through erythropoietin

a A patient, who you know to have received a renal transplant, asks what analgesic they might take to relieve mild pain after receiving a local anaesthetic

b In a patient who is going to receive a renal transplant, when is the most appropriate time to perform routine dental treatment?

c What is the most common cause of enamel loss in patients with chronic kidney disease?

d How does the kidney regulate blood pressure?

4 Risk markers in oral health assessment: From the list of options below, select the most likely answer. Each option may be used once, more than once, or not at all. Which of these factors is the most likely causative factor in the following scenarios?

A Radiotherapy

B Diabetes mellitus

C Gastric acid reflux

D Bruxism

E Smoking tobacco

F Pilocarpine tablets

G Hepatitis B

H The immunosuppressant drug cyclosporin A

a A patient attends with severely worn teeth but the silver amalgam fillings are raised above the level of the rest of the teeth

b A patient presents with a dry mouth and active caries. She stated that she had been treated recently for advanced squamous cell carcinoma of the head and neck complicated by severe oral mucositis

c This factor is associated with both oral cancer and increased severity of chronic periodontitis

d A patient attended the dental practice complaining of gingival hypertrophy. In her medical history she said she had hypertension and hypertriglyceridemia. She had recently received a kidney transplant

5 Eating disorders: From the list of options below, select the most likely answer. Each option may be used once, more than once, or not at all. What is the most likely diagnosis from the options listed below?

A Anorexia Nervosa

B Bulimia

C Pica

D Obesity

E Recreational use of amphetamines

F Hyperthyroidism

a A young female adult patient has a body mass index of 17.0. She wears large ill-fitting clothes. Her medical history reveals anaemia, and she admitted to using laxatives frequently

b A young patient who has a long standing tendency to eat dirt and sand

c A young female patient of nearly normal body weight has extensive dental caries. She reports eating large quantities of sugary foods followed by self-induced vomiting

d A male 15-year-old teenager has a body mass index above the 95% percentile for children of his age. He has non-alcoholic fatty liver disease, insulin resistance and low self-esteem

6 Which of the following conditions does not give rise to intrinsic staining of teeth?
A Tetracycline
B Internal resorption of the tooth crown
C Congenital erythropoietic porphyria
D Fluorosis
E Excessive consumption of tea and coffee

7 A patient requiring non-surgical periodontal treatment takes clopidogrel (an antiplatelet drug therapy). Which of the following is the best method of managing their care?
A This patient requires referral to a hospital care setting
B The clopidogrel medication should be stopped 12 hours before the treatment commences
C The INR should be assessed 12 hours prior to treatment
D Any bleeding can be managed by local haemostatic measures
E Extreme caution is needed if the blood platelets are between 150–450 × 10^9/L

8 Lichenoid mucosal reactions are more commonly seen adjacent to
A amalgam restorations
B gold inlays
C gold-porcelain crowns
D porcelain crowns
E glass ionomer restorations

9 When anaesthetising mandibular molar teeth with irreversible pulpitis, which of the following ancillary agents have been shown to improve the success rate of inferior alveolar nerve blocks (using lidocaine/adrenaline)?
A A buccal infiltration with 4% articaine and 1:100 000 adrenaline
B 30–50% nitrous oxide
C 600 mg Ibuprofen given 1 hour before anaesthesia
D 75 mg Indomethacin given 1 hour before anaesthesia
E All of the above

10 All healthcare workers should receive a hepatitis B immunisation. Choose one of the following options which best completes the sentence. For those who have not seroconverted after immunisation against hepatitis B

A operative dentistry should be avoided

B additional cross-infection measures are needed to prevent viral infection

C no special measures are required

D heavy duty gloves should be worn at all times

E there is an increased risk from other viral infections, for example from *Mycobacterium tuberculosis*

11 For each of the following patients select the most likely diagnosis. Each option may be used once, more than once, or not at all.

A Synovial chondromatosis

B Osseous ankylosis of the temporo-mandibular joint

C Condylar neck fracture

D Osteoarthritis of the temporo-mandibular joint

E Rheumatoid arthritis affecting the temporo-mandibular joint

F Hyperplasia of the right condyle

a Loose cartilaginous nodules increasing in size in the temporo-mandibular joint space. Joint movement is limited with pain and swelling

b The patient is unable to open their jaw. The normal structure of the temporo-mandibular joint appears absent on cone beam CT. There is a bony bridge between the mandibular ramus and the temporal bone

c The chin of the patient is deviated to the left side. The right side of the face appears elongated and this has been getting progressively more severe

d A patient complains of pain from the temporomandibular joint on movement of the mandible. The affected condyle is tender to palpation. A malocclusion is present with premature contact on the posterior teeth

e The patient has pain on opening with radiological evidence of erosion of the condyle and has a positive test for rheumatoid factor

12 Is there likely to be a substantial caries reduction benefit to a child from its mother taking prenatal fluoride supplements during pregnancy?

13 Bisphosphonates
  A act primarily to inhibit osteoblast function
  B are used in the prevention and treatment of osteoporosis
  C increase the risk of vertebral fracture in patients with osteoporosis
  D increase the rate of bone turnover
  E given intravenously, have a reduced risk of osteonecrosis of the jaw bone

14 Which of the following agents provides the most superior relief from moderate dental pain?
  A 400 mg Ibruprofen
  B 1000 mg paracetamol
  C 1000 mg aspirin

15 How soon after implant placement do immediate loading, early loading and conventional loading protocols take place?
  A At 2 weeks, 3–4 months and after 4 months, respectively
  B Within 1 week, 3–5 months and after 5 months, respectively
  C Within 1 week, 2–3 months and after 4 months, respectively
  D Within 1 week, 1 week to 2 months and after 2 months, respectively
  E Within 1 week, 5 months and after 6 months, respectively

16 Your patient has a history of recent deep vein thrombosis and is therefore taking warfarin. She has a stable international normalised ratio (INR) of 2.5. Would the INR be affected by the patient being prescribed topical miconazole for denture stomatitis?

17 Name two risk factors for alveolar osteitis ('dry socket'), a painful condition that can present a few days after a tooth extraction.

18 What are the main complications of dental relevance that might affect a patient with chronic renal disease?

19 Liver disease can give rise to excessive bleeding during surgery. What causes this excessive bleeding?
  A Impaired absorption of vitamin K
  B Abnormal platelet function and thrombocytopenia
  C Impaired production of clotting factors
  D Increased fibrinolysis
  E All of the above factors

20 Which of the following is an ester-type local anaesthetic?
  A Procaine
  B Lidocaine
  C Prilocaine
  D Articaine
  E Bupivacine

21 What is a typical presenting symptom of the Ramsay-Hunt syndrome?
  A Headache
  B Blisters in the hands
  C Unilateral facial paralysis
  D Swelling of the lips
  E Loss of speech

22 What is thought to be the cause of Bell's palsy?
  A Cerebrovascular ischaemia
  B Damage to the cortico-bulbar tract
  C Inflammation of the facial nerve in the stylomastoid foramen
  D Inflammation of the mandibular nerve in the stylomastoid foramen
  E None of the above

23 If a patient presents with symptoms of burning mouth syndrome, what investigations should be requested?
  A Blood glucose to exclude diabetes
  B Assessment of the quality of the patient's denture, especially whether freeway space is present
  C Swabs and smears to exclude candidal infection
  D Full blood count and haematinics screen (for serum vitamin B_{12}, serum folate, serum ferritin)
  E All the above

24 Giant cell arteritis is characterised by which of the following?
   A Sharp lancinating pain
   B Intense pain lasting for a few seconds
   C Unilateral throbbing pain in the area of the temple
   D Pain usually occurs bilaterally
   E The skin over the temple area is usually pain-free

25 In trigeminal neuralgia, which of the following options best describes the symptoms?
   A Sharp, intense pain lasting a few days
   B The pain can be initiated by gently stroking trigger zones in the neck
   C The pain can be alleviated with carbamazepine
   D There is often a tingling sensation that precedes the pain onset, followed by vesicle formation in the distribution of the nerve
   E The pain never undergoes spontaneous remission

26 The TNM classification system provides a method of tumour staging. Which of the following statements is correct?
   A The TNM classification assesses the size and location of the primary tumour invasion, the degree of regional lymph node involvement and whether distant metastases are present
   B Advanced stage disease is classified as stage I or II disease
   C Early stage disease is classified as stage III or IV disease
   D Stage I carcinoma of the oral cavity tends to be treated primarily by chemotherapy and radiation
   E The rate of occurrence of a second primary head and neck cancer is about 20% per year

27 According to the guidelines provided by the National Institute for Health and Care Excellence (2000), which of the following options would indicate that the impacted third molar should be removed?
   A All third molars should be removed prophylactically
   B The third molar has early enamel demineralisation
   C The patient has had one episode of mild pericoronitis
   D The impacted third molar is causing external resorption of the adjacent second molar
   E Plaque formation around the impacted wisdom tooth

28 You notice that a patient's dental panoramic tomogram has a generalised loss of lamina dura around the teeth. What medical condition might this indicate?

A Postmenopausal osteoporosis

B Paget's disease

C Cushing's syndrome

D Gardener's syndrome

E Autosomal dominant osteopetrosis

29 Which of the following options is correct?

A A dentist in the UK can use a private prescription to prescribe any medicine from the British National Formulary (BNF)

B In the UK, dental nurses may supply medicines without the prescription of a dentist

C Antimicrobial prophylaxis is recommended for the prevention of endocarditis in patients who are undergoing a tooth extraction

D Oral anticoagulants should be discontinued for 24 hours in the majority of patients requiring a single tooth extraction

E Amoxicillin can be used in patients who are allergic to penicillin

30 A tooth root is within the antrum. Which of the following surgical approaches is used to retrieve the root?

A Incision through the inferior conjunctival fornix

B Caldwell-Luc antrostomy

C Gillies' temporal approach

D A skin incision over the inferior orbital rim

E Preauricular approach

31 Which of the following options is correct? The oral manifestations of insulin-dependent diabetes may include

A a high caries rate

B an increased risk of squamous cell carcinoma

C oral candidosis

D leukolakia

E mucosal ulceration

32 Paterson-Kelly (or Plummer-Vinson) syndrome

A is associated with dysphagia

B affects mainly middle-aged men

C is mainly prevalent in equatorial Africa

D has no increased risk of carcinoma

E is a genetically inherited blood clotting disorder

33 Crohn's disease

A is an acute infection occurring on one occasion followed by life-long protection

B is characterised by chronic inflammation of the genito-urinary tract

C does not have a genetic component

D may include symptoms of labial swelling

E is characterised microscopically by necrotising granulomas

34 Salivary gland swelling may be a late complication of Sjogren's syndrome. Which is the correct option?

A Salivary gland swelling is caused by Raynaud's phenomenon

B Does not require investigation as it will get better

C Squamous cell carcinoma is a common late complication of Sjogren's disease

D Swelling may be due to mucosal candida infection

E Lymphoma may be present

35 Which option is correct? Monostotic fibrous dysplasia

A is characterised by skin pigmentation

B has bone lesions which radiographically have a well-defined corticated border

C is characterised by raised serum calcium

D most commonly has a 'ground-glass' radiographic pattern

E usually progresses into a polyostotic form of the disease affecting many bones

Answers

1 *Correct answer E*: With disc displacement with reduction, the disc is displaced anteriorly but is able to return to its normal position with further opening (when a click is heard). Crepitus (a crackling sound from the joint) indicates osteoarthritis. Locking of the jaw on opening indicates a diagnosis of TMJ disc displacement without reduction as the disc remains displaced and does not click back into place. De Leeuw *et al.* (1995) showed that even after 30 years of disc displacement with reduction, the radiographic changes to the joint were either absent or very slight (de Leeuw, R., Boering, G., Stegenga, B. and de Bont, L.G. Radiographic signs of temporomandibular joint osteoarthrosis and internal derangement 30 years after nonsurgical treatment. *Oral Surg. Oral Med. Oral Pathol. Oral Radiol. Endod.*, 1995, **79**: 382–92). The overbite and occlusion do not influence the prevalence of TMJ clicking (see Uhac, I., Kovac, Z., Vukovojac, S., Zuvić-Butorac, M., Grzić, R. and Delić, Z. The effect of occlusal relationships on the occurrence of sounds in the temporomandibular joint. *Coll. Antropol.*, 2002, **26**: 285–92).

2 **a** *Correct answer A*
   b *Correct answer D*: The noise from the joint was due to crepitation.
   c *Correct answer C*

3 **a** *Correct answer A*
   b *Correct answer D*
   c *Correct answer F*
   d *Correct answer G*
   The patient who has received a kidney transplant will be immunosuppressed and may also be receiving corticosteroids. Any dental infections should be avoided at this stage as they can be severe.

4 **a** *Correct answer C*
   b *Correct answer A*
   c *Correct answer E*
   d *Correct answer H*
   Pilocarpine tablets are used to treat the dry mouth symptoms of Sjogren's syndrome and head and neck radiotherapy. It is not clear from the dental literature whether patients with diabetes

are more prone to dental caries (see Sampaio, N., Mello, S. and Alves, C. Dental caries-associated risk factors and type 1 diabetes mellitus. *Pediatr. Endocrinol. Diabetes Metab.*, 2011, **17**: 152–7).

5 a *Correct answer A*
   b *Correct answer C*
   c *Correct answer B*
   d *Correct answer D*
   Hyperthyroidism typically involves weight loss, but hypothyroidism may cause weight gain and psychological changes. A higher incidence of hypothyroidism has been reported in patients with non-alcoholic fatty liver disease (see Pagadala, M.R., Zein, C.O., Dasarathy, S., Yerian, L.M., Lopez, R. and McCullough, A.J. Prevalence of hypothyroidism in nonalcoholic fatty liver disease. *Dig. Dis. Sci.*, 2012, **57**: 528–34).

6 *Correct answer E*: Tea and coffee are classified as agents causing extrinsic staining of teeth, not intrinsic staining. Fluoride and tetracycline affect the enamel colour during tooth development. Internal resorption is identified clinically as a pink spot. Congenital porphyria results in the circulation of red porphyrin pigments which stain the teeth a pink-brown colour.

7 *Correct answer D*: The normal platelet levels in the blood are 150–450 × 10^9/L. Discontinuing antiplatelet drugs may cause a rebound effect resulting in thromboembolic episodes. Bleeding following root planing and other non-surgical therapies can be easily controlled with applied pressure.

8 *Correct answer A*: In those patients with symptomatic lichenoid reactions adjacent to amalgam restorations, most patients derive some improvement by having these restorations replaced with another type of restoration material (see Dunsche, A., Kästel, I., Terheyden, H., Springer, I.N., Christophers, E. and Brasch, J. Oral lichenoid reactions associated with amalgam: improvement after amalgam removal. *Br. J. Dermatol.*, 2003, **148**: 70–6). Many of the patients whose lichenoid reactions improved by replacing their amalgam restorations had a negative patch test reaction to amalgam.

9 *Correct answer E*: Infection changes the pH of the tissues, reducing the number of local anaesthetic molecules which are lipid soluble. This reduces the efficacy of the local anaesthetic.

Stanley *et al.* (2012) showed that nitrous oxide may be given as an additional agent to increase the success rate of local anaesthetic when anaesthetising teeth with irreversible pulpitis (Stanley, W., Drum, M., Nusstein, J., Reader, A. and Beck, M. Effect of nitrous oxide on the efficacy of the inferior alveolar nerve block in patients with symptomatic irreversible pulpitis. *J. Endod.*, 2012, **38**: 565–9). Nitrous oxide provides a mild analgesic action. Matthews *et al.* (2009) described a 'modest success rate' of block anaesthesia when supplemented with a buccal infiltration of 4% articaine with 1:100 000 epinephrine (Matthews, R., Drum, M., Reader, A., Nusstein, J. and Beck, M. Articaine for supplemental buccal mandibular infiltration anesthesia in patients with irreversible pulpitis when the inferior alveolar nerve block fails. *J. Endod.*, 2009, **35**: 343–6).

Reducing the inflammation associated with irreversible pulpitis is effective in improving the success rate of anaesthesia. Parirokh *et al.* (2010) found that premedication with non-steroidal anti-inflammatory drugs were effective in improving the success rate of inferior alveolar nerve blocks for teeth with irreversible pulpitis (Parirokh, M., Ashouri, R., Rekabi, A.R. *et al.* The effect of premedication with ibuprofen and indomethacin on the success of inferior alveolar nerve block for teeth with irreversible pulpitis. *J. Endod.*, 2010, **36**: 1450–4).

10 *Correct answer C*: No special measures are required, because the routine, universal cross-infection control measures should provide sufficient protection. Rubber dam isolation with high volume aspiration should be used in routine dentistry to reduce spraying of blood, saliva or water aerosol and in conjunction with other protective barriers (e.g. plastic covers on surfaces, gloves, protective eyewear, and gowns). Masks and gloves should be changed routinely between patients.

Mycobacterium tuberculosis is a bacterium and not a virus. Those patients who are immunocompromised are more likely to be affected by tuberculosis than the general population.

11 a *Correct answer A*
   b *Correct answer B*
   c *Correct answer F*: Hyperplasia of the right condyle.
   d *Correct answer C*: With condylar neck fractures there is often deviation towards the fractured side (see Lindahl, L. Condylar fractures of the mandible. III. Positional changes of the chin. *Int. J. Oral Surg.*, 1977, **6**: 166–72).
   e *Correct answer E*: Changes in the occlusion (e.g. anterior open bite) may be present with severe condylar erosion. (For a detailed discussion of this topic see Bathi, R.J., Taneja, N. and Parveen, S. Rheumatoid arthritis of TMJ – a diagnostic dilemma? *Dent. Update*, 2004, **31**: 167–70, 172, 174).

12 *Correct answer*: No. Only a small amount of fluoride crosses the placental barrier.

13 *Correct answer B*

14 *Correct answer A*: According to a Cochrane review, 400 mg of ibruprofen is more effective than either 1000 mg of paracetamol or 1000 mg of aspirin (see Moore, R.A., Derry, S., McQuay, H.J. and Wiffen, P.J. Single dose oral analgesics for acute postoperative pain in adults. *Cochrane Database of Systematic Reviews* 2011, **Issue 9**: Art. No.: CD008659. DOI: 10.1002/14651858.CD008659.pub2).

15 *Correct answer D*: According to the systematic review by Esposito *et al.* (2013), immediate loading takes place within 1 week of implant placement and early loading between 1 week and 2 months after implant placement. Conventional protocols delay implant loading for at least 2 months (Esposito, M., Grusovin, M.G., Maghaireh, H. and Worthington, H.V. Interventions for replacing missing teeth: different times for loading dental implants. *Cochrane Database of Systematic Reviews* 2013, **Issue 3**: Art. No.: CD003878. DOI: 10.1002/14651858.CD003878.pub5).

16 *Correct answer*: Yes! Miconazole and fluconazole can cause drug interactions because they are absorbed. Miconazole can increase the INR if the warfarin dose is not decreased (see Kovac, M., Mitic, G. and Kovac, Z. Miconazole and nystatin used as topical antifungal drugs interact equally strongly with warfarin.

J. Clin. Pharm. Ther., 2012, Feb; **37(1):** 45–8. doi: 10.1111/ j.1365–2710.2011.01246.x. Epub 2011 Feb 17). The patient should be encouraged to clean the denture and store it in water overnight in a chlorhexidine solution. Chlorhexidine can also be used as an oral rinse. Denture trauma should be reduced by adjusting the occlusion and improving the fit of the dentures with tissue conditioner materials where necessary.

17 *Correct answer*: Risk factors include
1. Excessive surgical trauma
2. Smoking
3. Oral contraceptives
4. History of previous episodes of alveolar osteitis

18 *Correct answer*: Possible complications include
1. Bleeding
2. Infection
3. Drug toxicity
4. Anaemia
5. Hypertension
6. Hyperparathyridism

19 *Correct answer E*: Severe haemorrhage can result and it can be difficult to manage given the multiplicity of defects. Vitamin K is used in the liver's manufacture of the clotting factors II, VII, IX and X.

20 *Correct answer A*: Lidocaine, prilocaine, articaine and bupivacaine have amide links, but articaine is unusual in that it is classified as an amide local anaesthetic but has an ester link which when metabolised inactivates the molecule. Benzocaine and procaine are ester-type local anaesthetics.

21 *Correct answer C*: Ramsay-Hunt syndrome is caused by reactivation of herpes zoster infection of the geniculate ganglion (of the facial nerve). As well as the unilateral facial paralysis, other common symptoms include a loss of taste sensation, blisters in the ears and vertigo.

22 *Correct answer C*: Bell's palsy is caused by a lesion affecting the lower motoneurons of the facial nerve. The muscles of facial expression receive their motor supply from the facial nerve (not the mandibular nerve).

23 *Correct answer E*

24 *Correct answer C*

25 *Correct answer C*

26 *Correct answer A*: The actual risk of developing a second primary head and neck cancer is about 3–7% per year.

27 *Correct answer D*: The guidance states that removal of wisdom teeth should only be considered where the tooth is associated with pathology. Prophylactic removal of asymptomatic teeth should not be undertaken.

28 *Correct answer B*: Hyperparathyroidism and Paget's disease are associated with loss of the lamina dura. Postmenopausal osteoporosis is associated with a thinning of the inferior mandibular cortex, but the lamina dura has a normal appearance. Gardener's syndrome is associated with multiple osteomas and fibromas, sebaceous cysts and epidermoid cysts, but not generalised loss of the lamina dura. Gardener's syndrome is a sub-type of familial adenomatous polyposis and patients have an increased risk of malignant change in colon polyps. In Cushing's syndrome (caused by too high a level of glucocorticoid), patients have a high prevalence of osteoporosis with a partial thinning of the lamina dura. Hypophosphatasia (a genetic disease caused by a deficient activity of alkaline phosphatase) is associated with either a normal or thin lamina dura. The osteoclasts have a deficient function in autosomal dominant osteopetrosis and the bone is dense.

29 *Correct answer A*: Patient Group Directions (PGDs) are written instructions for the supply or administration of medicines to groups of patients who may not be individually identified before they present for treatment. According to the General Dental Council regulations, dental hygienists and dental therapists (not dental nurses) can independently supply or administer certain medicines for their patients' dental needs under Patient Group Directions. Oral anticoagulants should not be discontinued for patients undergoing tooth extraction due to the risk of thrombosis. The risk of significant bleeding is low in those with a stable INR of <4. The extraction should be performed as atraumatically as possible using oxidised cellulose (Surgicel) in the extraction socket to encourage haemostasis. Amoxicillin cannot be used in patients with an allergy to penicillin.

30 *Correct answer B*: An incision through the inferior orbital rim or through the inferior conjunctival fornix may be used to access the orbital floor following an orbital 'blow-out' fracture (see Harris, G.J. Orbital blow-out fractures: surgical timing and technique. *Eye*, 2006, **20**: 1207–12. doi:10.1038/sj.eye.6702384). A Gillies temporal approach is used to gain access to a fractured zygoma and allow it to be reduced. A Caldwell-Luc antrostomy allows a small window to be made in the anterior wall of the antrum and the root retrieved with Fickling's forceps. A preauricular approach is often used to gain access to the temporomandibular joint and would be an inappropriate surgical procedure for removing a root in the antrum.

31 *Correct answer C*: Oral candidosis can develop in poorly controlled diabetic patients.

32 *Correct answer A*: Paterson-Kelly syndrome is associated with a high incidence of post-cricoid carcinoma. It is more common in northern countries and affects more women than men. The dysphagia is associated with the post-cricoid region. Other features of the syndrome include iron deficiency anaemia and glossitis.

33 *Correct answer D*: Crohn's disease is characterised by chronic inflammation of the gastro-intestinal tract. It has a genetic component. The microscopic appearance is of non-necrotising granulomas, and the presence of a granuloma is not necessary for the diagnosis of Crohn's disease (see Geboes, K. What histologic features best differentiate Crohn's disease from ulcerative colitis? *Inflamm. Bowel. Dis.*, 2008, Oct; **14 Suppl 2:** S168–9).

34 *Correct answer E*: The swelling must be investigated as it may be due to a lymphoma. These patients have an increased incidence of lymphoma (37.5 times greater than the general population according to a study by Lazarus *et al.* in 2006 (Lazarus, M.N., Robinson, D., Mak, V., Møller, H. and Isenberg, D.A. Incidence of cancer in a cohort of patients with primary Sjogren's syndrome. *Rheumatology* (Oxford), 2006, Aug; **45(8):** 1012–5). Also, there was no increased incidence of other cancers in patients with Sjogren's disease. They may experience Raynaud's phenomenon, which is a vasomotor disturbance of the fingers.

35 *Correct answer D*: Monostotic fibrous dysplasia does not progress into a polyostotic form of the disease. Radiographically, monostotic fibrous dysplasia has no defined bony margin. Albright's syndrome describes polyostotic fibrous dysplasia with skin pigmentation and precocious female puberty.

CHAPTER 12

Paediatric dentistry, public dental health and orthodontics

Questions

1 Which of the following is not included in the treatment a dental therapist can provide for patients in general dental practice in the UK?
   A Performing pulpotomies on primary teeth
   B Direct restorations on permanent teeth
   C Indirect restorations on permanent teeth
   D Care of implants and treating peri-implant disease
   E Prescribe radiographs

2 What is the Hall technique?
   A A method of providing painless local anaesthetic
   B A patient management technique
   C A patient acclimitisation technique
   D Uses preformed nickel-chrome crowns cemented over the carious tooth
   E Involves complete removal of caries from the tooth under local anaesthetic

3 Vital pulp therapy for the primary tooth involves placing over the pulp chamber cotton wool dampened with
   A Formocresol
   B Ferric sulphate to arrest bleeding. This is then removed and a zinc-oxide eugenol dressing is placed in the pulp chamber.

Review Questions for Dentistry, First Edition. Hugh Devlin.
© 2017 John Wiley & Sons, Ltd. Published 2017 by John Wiley & Sons, Ltd.
Companion Website: www.wiley.com/go/devlin/review_questions_for_dentistry

   C Sodium hypochlorite solution
   D Beechwood creostote
   E Ledermix

4 Following trauma to an upper incisor of a patient, the tooth undergoes lateral luxation (displacement). What treatment would you advise?
   A Stabilise the tooth for 6 days and examine the tooth radiographically after this interval
   B Immediately treat the tooth endodontically if it is non-responsive to vitality testing
   C Reposition the tooth under local anaesthesia and stabilise it for 4 weeks
   D Wait for the tooth to re-erupt
   E No treatment is usually recommended other than to recommend a soft diet

5 A 12-year-old child attends with a mid-root fractured upper central incisor following trauma. You decide to reposition the tooth because it is slightly displaced, but how long would you recommend splinting the tooth using a composite or wire/composite splint?
   A 4 days
   B 4 weeks
   C 4 months
   D 6 months
   E Permanently

6 The most sensitive method of diagnosing enamel demineralisation in the occlusal surface of a lower first molar involves
   A using bitewing radiography
   B drying the tooth followed by careful visual examination
   C probing the area carefully
   D using panoramic radiography
   E brushing the tooth to see whether it is staining rather than caries that is present

7 A lower first primary molar requires to be anaesthetised with local anaesthetic prior to minor routine conservation in a

cooperative child. Which procedure is the first choice to anaesthetise the tooth?

A Inter-papillary injection
B Buccal infiltration
C Inferior alveolar nerve block
D Intra-septal injection
E Lingual infiltration

8 A teenage patient presents with an instanding upper central incisor and requests its correction orthodontically. Which of the following are necessary if the anterior crossbite is to be corrected with a simple removable appliance?

A Adequate mesio-distal space should be present for the new position of the central incisor in the arch
B The apex of the central incisor should be close to its final position
C After correction, an overbite will be present to maintain the tooth position
D The other teeth are in an ideal relationship
E All of the above should be present

9 Which of the following statements is correct?

A A replanted avulsed upper tooth is less likely to become ankylosed if the tooth is replanted within 5 minutes
B The tooth always becomes ankylosed so replantation is rarely viable
C If the tooth becomes ankylosed, the further vertical development of the alveolar ridge is not affected during continued growth of the child.
D If the ideal conditions to prevent ankylosis are not present, the tooth should not be implanted
E Whether a tooth becomes ankylosed depends on the blood supply to the pulp of the implanted tooth

Answers

1 *Correct answer C*

2 *Correct answer D*: The Hall technique involves using a preformed crown to seal the carious tooth.

3 *Correct answer B*: If bleeding is excessive, cotton wool dampened with ferric sulphate may need to be sealed into the pulp chamber between appointments. Normally, bleeding stops within 2 to 3 minutes and the pulpal canal orifices can be covered with either (a) setting calcium hydroxide cement and zinc oxide eugenol dressing or (b) a zinc oxide dressing and a preformed crown. Formocresol is not considered safe; however, a recent paper reviewed the evidence and found that the amount of formaldehyde released from formocresol during the few minutes exposure in a pulpotomy was small and unlikely to pose any health concerns (see Athanassiadis, B., George, G.A., Abbott, P.V. and Wash, L.J. A review of the effects of formaldehyde release from endodontic materials. *Int. Endod. J.*, 2015, **48:** 829–38).

4 *Correct answer C*: A 4-week stabilisation period is usually required because the alveolar bone is usually fractured. With vitality testing, the tooth is often non-responsive but the risk of true pulpal necrosis is dependent on whether the root apices are closed and whether there is any other associated fracture of the tooth.

5 *Correct answer B*: A stabilisation period of 4 weeks is usually recommended. The exception is where the patient has a cervical root fracture and in that situation the stabilisation period should be 4 months. The tooth should be examined clinically and radiographically at 2, 4, 6 and 12 month intervals. At about 4 months, should the tooth show radiographic signs of non-vitality (radiolucency adjacent to the fracture line) and fail to respond to vitality tests, the coronal fragment should be endodontically treated and filled to the fracture line.

6 *Correct answer B*: Bitewing radiographs can be useful in diagnosing interproximal and occult caries, but the thickness of enamel would be likely to obscure enamel demineralisation. Early enamel demineralisation has an opaque, chalky white appearance.

7 *Correct answer B*: Intra-septal injections may be used to supplement a buccal infiltration.

8 *Correct answer E*

9 *Correct answer A*: It is not inevitable that a replanted tooth will become ankylosed, especially if reimplanted within a few minutes. In the emergency situation, replanting an avulsed tooth allows time for construction of a treatment plan between specialist colleagues, even when the ideal conditions are not met. The main factor that prevents ankylosis is whether a viable periodontal ligament remains on the implanted tooth, not a vital pulp. If a tooth becomes ankylosed it can cause a reduced alveolar ridge development during the adolescent growth spurt. To prevent this scenario, some advocate decoronating the ankylosed tooth to allow alveolar bone to growth over the resorbing root. If the tooth starts to become infra-occluded by 2 mm or more and the patient is at the start of the growth spurt then decoronation has the best chance of success in preventing an alveolar defect.

Further reading

Al-Ani, Z., Gray, R.J., Davies, S.J., Sloan, P. and Glenny, A.M. Stabilization splint therapy for the treatment of temporomandibular myofascial pain: a systematic review. *J. Dent. Educ.*, 2005, **69**: 1242–50.

Alapati, S.B., Brantley, W.A., Iijima, M., Clark, W.A., Kovarik, L., Buie, C., Liu, J. and Ben Johnson, W. Metallurgical characterization of a new nickel-titanium wire for rotary endodontic instruments. *J. Endod.*, 2009, **35**: 1589–93.

Alomari, Q.D., Reinhardt, J.W. and Boyer, D.B. Effect of liners on cusp deflection and gap formation in composite restorations. *Op. Dent.*, 2001, **26**: 406–41.

Athanassiadis, B., George, G.A., Abbott, P.V. and Wash, L.J. A review of the effects of formaldehyde release from endodontic materials. *Int. Endod. J.*, 2015, **48**: 829–38.

Baljoon. M., Natto, S. and Bergström, J. Long-term effect of smoking on vertical periodontal bone loss. *J. Clin. Periodontol.*, 2005, Jul; **32(7)**: 789–97.

Bathi, R.J., Taneja, N. and Parveen, S. Rheumatoid arthritis of TMJ – a diagnostic dilemma? *Dent. Update*, 2004, **31**: 167–70, 172, 174.

Biswas, M., Mazumdar, D. and Neyogi, A. Non-surgical perforation repair by mineral trioxide aggregate under dental operating microscope. *J. Conserv. Dent.*, 2011, **14**: 83–5.

Bogen, G., Kim, J.S. and Bakland, L.K. Direct pulp capping with mineral trioxide aggregate: an observational study. *J. Am. Dent. Assoc.*, 2008, **139**: 305–15.

Burke, F.J. Resin-retained bridges: fibre-reinforced versus metal. *Dent. Update*, 2008, **35**: 521–2, 524–6.

Burke, F.J.T. and Lucarotti, P.S.K. Ten-year outcome of crowns placed within the General Dental Services in England and Wales. *J. Dentistry*, 2009, **37**: 12–24.

Campos, M.L., Corrêa, M.G., Júnior, F.H., Casati, M.Z., Sallum, E.A. and Sallum, A.W. Cigarette smoke inhalation increases the alveolar bone loss caused by primary occlusal trauma in a rat model. *J. Periodont. Res.*, 2014, Apr; **49(2)**: 179–85.

Carlsson, G.E. Critical review of some dogmas in prosthodontics. *J. Prosthodont. Res.*, 2009, **53**: 3–10.

Carter, R.B. and Keen, E.N. The intramandibular course of the inferior alveolar nerve. *J. Anat.*, 1971, **108(Pt 3)**: 433–40.

Cheung, G.S. and Stock, C.J. *In vitro* cleaning ability of root canal irrigants with and without endosonics. *Int. Endod. J.*, 1993, **26**: 334–43.

Corbet, E.F. Oral diagnosis and treatment planning: Part 3: Periodontal disease and assessment of risk. *Br. Dent. J.*, 2012, **213**: 111–21. doi: 10.1038/sj.bdj.2012.666.

Review Questions for Dentistry, First Edition. Hugh Devlin.
© 2017 John Wiley & Sons, Ltd. Published 2017 by John Wiley & Sons, Ltd.
Companion Website: www.wiley.com/go/devlin/review_questions_for_dentistry

Cortellini, P. and Pini Prato, G. Coronally advanced flap and combination therapy for root coverage. Clinical strategies based on scientific evidence and clinical experience. *Periodontol. 2000*, 2012, **59:** 158–84.

Culwick, P.F., Howell, P.G. and Faigenblum, M.J. The size of occlusal rest seats prepared for removable partial dentures. *Br. Dent. J.,* 2000, **189:** 318–22.

Dalton, B.C., Ørstavik, D., Philips, C., Pettiette, M. and Trope, M. Bacterial reduction with nickel-titanium rotary instrumentation. *J. Endod.,* 1998, **24:** 763–7.

Dang, N., Meshram, G.K. and Mittal, R.K. Effects of designs of Class 2 preparations on resistance of teeth to fracture. *Indian J. Dent. Res.,* 1997, **8:** 90–4.

Dastmalchi, N., Kazemi, Z., Hashemi, S., Peters, O.A. and Jafarzadeh, H. Definition and endodontic treatment of dilacerated canals: a survey of Diplomates of the American Board of Endodontics. *J. Contemp. Dent. Pract.,* 2011, **12:** 8–13.

Delivanis, P.D., Snowden, R.B. and Doyle, R.J. Localization of blood-borne bacteria in instrumented unfilled root canals. *Oral Surg. Oral Med. Oral Pathol.,* 1981, **52:** 430–2.

de Leeuw, R., Boering, G., Stegenga, B. and de Bont, L.G. Radiographic signs of temporomandibular joint osteoarthrosis and internal derangement 30 years after nonsurgical treatment. *Oral Surg. Oral Med. Oral Pathol. Oral Radiol. Endod.,* 1995, **79:** 382–92.

De Munck, J., Van Landuyt, K., Peumans, M., Poitevin, A., Lambrechts, P., Braem, M. and Van Meerbeek, B. A critical review of the durability of adhesion to tooth tissue: methods and results. *J. Dent. Res.,* 2005, **84:** 118–32.

Derdilopoulou, F.V., Zantner, C., Neumann, K. and Kielbassa, A.M. Evaluation of visual and spectrophotometric shade analyses: a clinical comparison of 3758 teeth. *Int. J. Prosthodont.,* 2007, **20:** 414–6.

Dunsche, A., Kästel, I., Terheyden, H., Springer, I.N., Christophers, E. and Brasch, J. Oral lichenoid reactions associated with amalgam: improvement after amalgam removal. *Br. J. Dermatol.,* 2003, **148:** 70–6.

Esposito, M., Grusovin, M.G., Maghaireh, H. and Worthington, H.V. Interventions for replacing missing teeth: different times for loading dental implants. Cochrane Database of Systematic Reviews 2013, Issue 3. Art. No.: CD003878. DOI: 10.1002/14651858.CD003878.pub5.

European Society of Endodontology. Quality guidelines for endodontic treatment: consensus report of the European Society of Endodontology. *Int. Endod. J.,* 2006, **39:** 921–30.

Fedorowicz, Z., Nasser, M. and Wilson. N. Adhesively-bonded versus non-bonded amalgam restorations for dental caries. *Cochrane Database of Systematic Reviews 2009*, **Issue 4:** Art. No.: CD007517. DOI: 10.1002/14651858.CD007517.pub2.

Feres, M., Soares, G.M., Mendes, J.A., Silva, M.P., Faveri, M., Teles, R., Socransky, S.S. and Figueiredo, L.C. Metronidazole alone or with amoxicillin as adjuncts to non-surgical treatment of chronic periodontitis: a 1-year double-blinded, placebo-controlled, randomised clinical trial. *J. Clin. Periodont.,* 2012, **39:** 1149–58.

Fernandes, A.S. and Dessai, G.S. Factors affecting the fracture resistance of post-core reconstructed teeth: a review. *Int. J. Prosthodont.,* 2001, **14:** 355–63.

Firatli, E. The relationship between clinical periodontal status and insulin-dependent diabetes mellitus. Results after 5 years. *J Periodontol.*, 1997, **68**(2): 136–40.

Fukushima, H., Yamamoto, K., Hirohata, K., Sagawa, H., Leung, K.P. and Walker, C.B. Localization and identification of root canal bacteria in clinically asymptomatic periapical pathosis. *J. Endod.*, 1990, **16**: 534–8.

Geboes, K. What histologic features best differentiate Crohn's disease from ulcerative colitis? *Inflamm. Bowel. Dis.*, 2008, Oct; **14 Suppl** 2: S168–9.

Genco, R.J., Ho, A.W., Kopman, J., Grossi, S.G., Dunford, R.G. and Tedesco, L.A. Models to evaluate the role of stress in periodontal disease. *Ann. Periodontol.*, 1998, **3**: 288–302.

Gomez, J., Pretty, I.A., Santarpia, R.P. 3rd, Cantore, B., Rege, A., Petrou, I. and Ellwood, R.P. Quantitative light-induced fluorescence to measure enamel remineralization *in vitro*. *Caries Res.*, 2014, **48**: 223–7.

Hamp, S.E., Nyman, S. and Lindhe, J. Periodontal treatment of multirooted teeth. Results after 5 years. *J. Clin. Periodontol.* 1975. **2**: 126–35.

Hancock, H.H. 3rd, Sigurdsson, A., Trope, M. and Moiseiwitsch, J. Bacteria isolated after unsuccessful endodontic treatment in a North American population. *Oral Surg. Oral Med. Oral Pathol. Oral Radiol. Endod.*, 2001, **91**: 579–86.

Harris, G.J. Orbital blow-out fractures: surgical timing and technique. *Eye*, 2006, **20**: 1207–12. doi:10.1038/sj.eye.6702384.

Hassanien, E.E., Hashem, A. and Chalfin, H. Histomorphometric study of the root apex of mandibular premolar teeth: an attempt to correlate working length measured with electronic and radiograph methods to various anatomic positions in the apical portion of the canal. *J. Endod.*, 2008, **34**: 408–12.

Hosey, M.T. UK National Clinical Guidelines in Paediatric Dentistry. Managing anxious children: the use of conscious sedation in paediatric dentistry. *Int. J. Paediatr. Dent.*, 2002, *Sept;* **12**(5): 359–72.

Howdle, M.D., Fox, K. and Youngson, C.C. An *in vitro* study of coronal microleakage around bonded amalgam coronal-radicular cores in endodontically treated molar teeth *Quintessence Int.*, 2002, **33**: 22–9.

International Workshop for a Classification of Periodontal Diseases and Conditions. Papers. Oak Brook, Illinois, 30 October–2 November 1999. *Ann. Periodontol.*, 1999, **4i**: 1–112.

Isa, Z.M. and Abdulhadi, L.M. Relationship of maxillary incisors in complete dentures to the incisive papilla. *J. Oral Sci.*, 2012, **54**(2): 159–63.

Izu, K.H., Thomas, S.J., Zhang, P., Izu, A.E. and Michalek, S. Effectiveness of sodium hypochlorite in preventing inoculation of periapical tissues with contaminated patency files. *J. Endod.*, 2004, **30**: 92–4.

Kovac, M., Mitic, G. and Kovac, Z. Miconazole and nystatin used as topical antifungal drugs interact equally strongly with warfarin. *J. Clin. Pharm. Ther.*, 2012, Feb; **37**(1): 45–8. doi: 10.1111/j.1365–2710.2011.01246.x. Epub 2011 Feb 17).

Lang, N.P., Berglundh, T., Heitz-Mayfield, L.J., Pjetursson, B.E., Salvi, G.E. and Sanz, M. Consensus statements and recommended clinical procedures regarding implant survival and complications. *Int. J. Oral Maxillofac. Implants*, 2004, **9 Suppl**: 150–4.

Lazarus, M.N., Robinson, D., Mak, V., Møller, H. and Isenberg, D.A. Incidence of cancer in a cohort of patients with primary Sjogren's syndrome. *Rheumatology (Oxford)*, 2006, Aug; **45**(8): 1012–5.

Lin, H.P., Wang, Y.P., Chen, H.M., Cheng, S.J., Sun, A. and Chiang, C.P. A clinicopathological study of 338 dentigerous cysts. *J. Oral. Pathol. Med.*, 2013, **42**(6): 462–7.

Lindahl, L. Condylar fractures of the mandible. III. Positional changes of the chin. *Int. J. Oral Surg.*, 1977, **6**: 166–72.

Loizeaux, A.D. and Devos, B.J. Inferior alveolar nerve anomaly. *J. Hawaii Dent. Assoc.*, 1981, **12**: 10–11.

López, N.J., Gamonal, J.A. and Martinez, B. Repeated metronidazole and amoxicillin treatment of periodontitis. A follow-up study. *J. Periodontol.*, 2000, **71**: 79–89.

Loutfy, M.R. and Walmsley, S.L. Salvage antiretroviral therapy in HIV infection. *Opin. Pharmacother.*, 2002, **3**: 81–90.

Makedonas, D., Odman, A. and Hansen, K. Management of root resorption in a large orthodontic clinic. *Swed. Dent. J.*, 2009, **33**: 173–80.

Marotta, P.S., Fontes, T.V., Armada, L., Lima, K.C., Rôças, I.N. and Siqueira, J.F. Jr., Type 2 diabetes mellitus and the prevalence of apical periodontitis and endodontic treatment in an adult Brazilian population. *J. Endod.*, 2012, **38**: 297–300.

Martinho, F.C., Gomes, A.P., Fernandes, A.M., Ferreira, N.S., Endo, M.S., Freitas, L.F. and Camões, I.C. Clinical comparison of the effectiveness of single-file reciprocating systems and rotary systems for removal of endotoxins and cultivable bacteria from primarily infected root canals. *J. Endod.*, 2014, **40**: 625–9.

Matthews, D.C. The relationship between diabetes and periodontal disease. *J. Can. Dent. Assoc.*, 2002, **68**(3): 161–4.

Matthews, R., Drum, M., Reader, A., Nusstein, J. and Beck, M. Articaine for supplemental buccal mandibular infiltration anesthesia in patients with irreversible pulpitis when the inferior alveolar nerve block fails. *J. Endod.*, 2009, **35**: 343–6.

Moore, R.A., Derry, S., McQuay, H.J. and Wiffen, P.J. Single dose oral analgesics for acute postoperative pain in adults. *Cochrane Database of Systematic Reviews* 2011, **Issue 9**: Art. No.: CD008659. DOI: 10.1002/14651858.CD008659.pub2.

Morgan, L.F. and Montgomery, S. An evaluation of the crown-down pressureless technique. *J. Endod.*, 1984, **10**: 491–8.

Nasser, M. Evidence summary: which dental liners under amalgam restorations are more effective in reducing postoperative sensitivity? *Brit. Dent. J.*, 2011, **210**: 533–7.

Nathanson, D. and Parra, C. Bleaching vital teeth: a review and clinical study. *Compend. Contin. Educ. Dent.*, 1987, **8**: 490–7.

Nayyar, A., Walton, R.E. and Leonard, L.A. An amalgam coronal-radicular dowel and core technique for endodontically treated posterior teeth. *J. Prosthet. Dent.*, 1980, **43**: 511–5.

Needleman, H.L., Allred, E., Bellinger, D., Leviton, A., Rabinowitz, M. and Iverson, K. Antecedents and correlates of hypoplastic enamel defects of primary incisors. *Pediatr. Dent.*, 1992, **14**(3): 158–66.

Nishikawa, S., Nagata, T., Morisaki, I., Oka, T. and Ishida, H. Pathogenesis of drug-induced gingival overgrowth. A review of studies in the rat model. *J. Periodontol.*, 1996, **67**: 463–71.

Nyman, S., Lindhe, J., Karring, T. and Rylander, H. New attachment following surgical treatment of human periodontal disease. *J. Clin. Periodontol.*, 1982, **9**: 290–6.

Pagadala, M.R., Zein, C.O., Dasarathy, S., Yerian, L.M., Lopez, R. and McCullough, A.J. Prevalence of hypothyroidism in nonalcoholic fatty liver disease. *Dig. Dis. Sci.*, 2012, **57**: 528–34.

Parirokh, M., Ashouri, R., Rekabi, A.R., Nakhaee, N., Pardakhti, A., Askarifard, S. and Abbott, P.V. The effect of premedication with ibuprofen and indomethacin on the success of inferior alveolar nerve block for teeth with irreversible pulpitis. *J. Endod.*, 2010, **36**: 1450–4.

Paris, S., Meyer-Lueckel, H. and Kielbassam A.M. Resin infiltration of natural caries lesions. *J. Dent. Res.*, 2007, **86**: 662–6.

Parker, M.H., Calverley, M.J., Gardner, F.M. and Gunderson, R.B. New guidelines for preparation taper. *J. Prosthodont.*, 1993, Mar; **2(1)**: 61–6.

Peeters, H.H., Suardita, K. and Setijanto, D. Prevalence of a second canal in the mesiobuccal root of permanent maxillary first molars from an Indonesian population. *J. Oral. Sci.*, 2011, **53**: 489–94.

Pontius, V., Pontius, O., Braun, A., Frankenberger, R. and Roggendorf, M.J. Retrospective evaluation of perforation repairs in 6 private practices. *J. Endod.*, 2013, **39**: 1346–58.

Poulsen, S., Errboe, M., Lescay Mevil, Y. and Glenny, A.M. Potassium-containing toothpastes for dentine hypersensitivity. *Cochrane Database of Systematic Reviews* 2006, **Issue 3**: Art. No.: CD001476. DOI: 10.1002/14651858.CD001476.pub2.

Pratten, D.H. and McDonald, N.J. Comparison of radiographic and electronic working lengths. *J. Endod.*, 1996, **22**: 173–6.

Preus, H.R., Gunleiksrud, T.M., Sandvik, L., Gjermo, P. and Baelum, V. A randomised, double-masked clinical trial comparing four periodontitis treatment strategies: 1-year clinical results. *J. Periodontol.*, 2013, **84**: 1075–86.

Quality guidelines for endodontic treatment: consensus report of the European Society of Endodontology. *Int. Endod. J.*, 2006, **39**: 921–30.

Rams, T.E., Degenerm, J.E. and van Winkelhoff, A.J. Antibiotic resistance in human chronic periodontitis microbiota. *J. Periodontol.*, 2014, **85**: 160–9.

Rasimick, B.J., Wan, J., Musikant, B.L. and Deutsch, A.S. A review of failure modes in teeth restored with adhesively luted endodontic dowels. *J. Prosthod.*, 2010, **19**: 639–46.

Renton, T., Hankins, M., Sproate, C. and McGurk, M. A randomised controlled clinical trial to compare the incidence of injury to the inferior alveolar nerve as a result of coronectomy and removal of mandibular third molars. *Br. J. Oral Maxillofac. Surg.*, 2005, Feb; **43(1)**: 7–12.

Ricucci, D., Siqueira, J.F. Jr, Bate, A.L. and Pitt Ford, T.R. Histologic investigation of root canal-treated teeth with apical periodontitis: a retrospective study from twenty-four patients. *J. Endod.*, 2009, **35**: 493–502.

Roberts, J.A., Drage, N.A., Davies, J. and Thomas, D.W. Effective dose from cone beam CT examinations in dentistry. *Br. J. Radiol.*, 2009, **82**: 35–40.

Robinson, P. and Lee, J.W. The use of real time video magnification for the pre-clinical teaching of crown preparations. *Br. Dent. J.*, 2001, **190:** 506–10.

Sampaio, N., Mello, S. and Alves, C. Dental caries-associated risk factors and type 1 diabetes mellitus. *Pediatr. Endocrinol. Diabetes Metab.*, 2011, **17:** 152–7.

Siqueira, J.F. Jr, Rôças, I.N., Riche, F.N. and Provenzano, J.C. Clinical outcome of the endodontic treatment of teeth with apical periodontitis using an antimicrobial protocol. *Oral Surg. Oral Med. Oral Pathol. Oral Radiol. Endod.*, 2008, **106:** 757–62.

Slaus, G. and Bottenberg, P. A survey of endodontic practice amongst Flemish dentists. *Int. Endod. J.*, 2002, **35:** 759–67.

Smales, R.J. and Hawthorne, W.S. Long-term survival of extensive amalgams and posterior crowns. *J. Dent.*, 1997, **25:** 225–7.

Souza, E.M., Bretas, R.T., Cenci, M.S., Maia-Filho, E.M. and Bonetti-Filho, I. Periapical radiographs overestimate root canal wall thickness during post space preparation. *Int. Endo. J.*, 2008, **41:** 658–63.

Stanley, W., Drum, M., Nusstein, J., Reader, A. and Beck, M. Effect of nitrous oxide on the efficacy of the inferior alveolar nerve block in patients with symptomatic irreversible pulpitis. *J. Endod.*, 2012, **38:** 565–9.

Stoltze, K. Concentration of metronidazole in periodontal pockets after application of a metronidazole 25% dental gel. *Clin. Periodontol.*, 1992, **19(9 Pt 2):** 698–701.

Torabinejad, M., Kettering, J.D., McGraw, J.C., Cummings, R.R., Dwyer, T.G. and Tobias, T.S. Factors associated with endodontic interappointment emergencies of teeth with necrotic pulps. *J. Endod.*, 1988, **14:** 261–6.

Tsesis, I., Faivishevsky, V., Fuss, Z. and Zukerman, O. Flare-ups after endodontic treatment: a meta-analysis of literature. *J. Endod.*, 2008, **34:** 1177–81.

Uçtaşli, M.B. and Tinaz, A.C. Microleakage of different types of temporary restorative materials used in endodontics. *J. Oral. Sci.*, 2000, **42:** 63–7.

Uhac, I., Kovac, Z., Vukovojac, S., Zuvić-Butorac, M., Grzić, R. and Delić, Z. The effect of occlusal relationships on the occurrence of sounds in the temporomandibular joint. *Coll. Antropol.*, 2002, **26:** 285–92.

Van Nieuwenhuysen, J.P., D'Hoore, W.D., Carvalho, J. and Qvist, V. Long-term evaluation of extensive restorations in permanent teeth. *J. Dent.*, 2003, **31:** 395–405.

Versluis, A., Tantbirojn, D., Lee, M.S., Tu, L.S. and DeLong, R. Can hygroscopic expansion compensate polymerization shrinkage? Part I: Deformation of restored teeth. *Dent. Mat.*, 2011, **27:** 126–33.

Wang. J., Lin, J., Seliger, A., Gil, M., da Silva, J.D. and Ishhikawa-Nagai, S. Color effects of gingiva on cervical regions of all-ceramic crowns. *J. Esthet. Restor. Dent.*, 2013, **25:** 254–62.

Webber, R.T., del Rio, C.E., Brady, J.M. and Segall R.O. Sealing quality of a temporary filling material. *Oral. Surg. Oral Med. Oral Pathol.*, 1978, Jul; **46(1):** 123–30.

Wedenberg, C. and Lindskog, S. Evidence for a resorption inhibitor in dentine. *Eur. J. Oral. Sci.*, 1987, **95:** 205–11.

White, D.A., Tsakos, G., Pitts, N.B., Fuller, E., Douglas, G.V., Murray, J.J. and, Steele, J.G. Adult Dental Health Survey 2009: common oral health conditions and their impact on the population. *Br. Dent. J.*, 2012, **213:** 567–72.

Wiegand, T. and Attin, T. Treatment of proximal caries lesions by tunnel restorations. *Dent. Mat.*, 2007, **23:** 1461–7.

Wolcott, J., Ishley, D., Kennedy, W., Johnson, S. and Minnich, S. Clinical investigation of second mesiobuccal canals in endodontically treated and retreated maxillary molars. *J. Endod.*, 2002, **28:** 477–9.

Wu, M.K., van der Sluis, L.W. and Wesselink, P.R. The capability of two hand instrumentation techniques to remove the inner layer of dentine in oval canals. *Int. Endod. J.*, 2003, **36:** 218–24.

Yadav, M., Godge, P., Meghana, S.M. and Kulkarni, S.R. Compound odontoma. *Contemp. Clin. Dent.*, 2012, Apr; **3(Suppl 1):** S13–5.

Yingling, N.M., Byrne, B.E. and Hartwell, G.R. Antibiotic use by members of the American Association of Endodontists in the year 2000; report of a national survey. *J. Endod.*, 2002, **28:** 396–404.

Yoon, S.S., Cheong, C., Preisser, J. Jr, Jun, S., Chang, B.M. and Wright, R.F. Measurement of total occlusal convergence of three different tooth preparations in four different planes by dental students. *J. Prosthet. Dent.*, 2014, **pii:** S0022–3913(14)00099–7. doi: 10.1016/j.prosdent.2014.01.021.

Yuan, Y., L'italien, G., Mukherjee, J. and Iloeje, U.H. Determinants of discontinuation of initial highly active antiretroviral therapy regimens in a US HIV-infected patient cohort. *HIV Med.*, 2006, **7:** 156–62.

http://www.bsperio.org.uk/publications/downloads/39_143748_bpe2011.pdf

https://www.icdas.org/uploads/ICDAS%20Criteria%20Manual%20Revised%202009_2.pdf

Index

Abfraction lesions, 101, 135
Abutment, 25–26, 58, 130, 133
Access cavity, 3–5, 51–52, 54
Altered cast technique, 130, 133
Alveolar osteitis ("dry socket"), 158
Amalgam, 19–22, 51, 97, 99–100,
    102–103, 107, 119, 155–156
Angular bony defect, 79
Anterior guidance, 118, 123, 135
Antibiotics, 12
Apex locator, 3
Apexification, 6
Apical transportation, 4
Articulator, 122, 130–131, 135
Atraumatic restorative treatment
    (ART), 99

Balanced force technique, 52
Basic Periodontal Examination (BPE),
    11, 76, 83
Bell's palsy, 159
Biofilm, 75, 77, 119
Biological width, 80, 124
Biometric guidelines, 27, 134
Bisphosphonates, 158
Bleaching of teeth, 60, 125–126
Bridge, 26, 58, 127, 131
BULL rule, 132
Burning mouth syndrome, 159

CAD/CAM, 21
Caries-detector dye, 99
Cavity design, 20, 106
Cement, 19, 20, 121, 124, 127, 137
Cephalometry, 42
Ceramic inlays, 21

Chlorhexidine, 5, 58, 77
Chronic periodontitis, 12–13, 25, 53,
    76, 78, 84, 155
Cleft lip, 43
Clopidogrel, 156
Combination syndrome, 132
Coagulation of blood, 34
Complete dentures, 25, 28, 131–132,
    134, 136
Compound odontome, 36
Cone beam computed tomography
    (CBCT), 5, 55, 57
Configuration factor, 106
Copy (or replica) denture technique,
    136
Coronectomy, 36
Crohn's disease, 162
Crown-down technique, 52
Crowns, 27, 118, 121, 123, 135, 156,
    171

Dentigerous cyst, 36
Dentine, 20–21, 52–54, 58, 97–103,
    106, 118, 120, 125–127, 137
Dentine hypersensitivity, 106
Denture clasp design, 126, 128, 130,
    133
Denture connector, 127–128, 130
Denture stomatitis, 25, 28, 158
Diabetes, 13, 53, 78, 86, 87, 154, 159,
    161
Disinfection, 26, 60

Eating disorders, 40, 155
Endodontic access cavity, 5

Review Questions for Dentistry, First Edition. Hugh Devlin.
© 2017 John Wiley & Sons, Ltd. Published 2017 by John Wiley & Sons, Ltd.
Companion Website: www.wiley.com/go/devlin/review_questions_for_dentistry

Erosion of teeth, 26, 135
Every denture, 133

Fibrous dysplasia, 162
Fibrous epulis, 78
Fluoride, 40–42, 99, 104, 118, 125, 158
Fovea palatinae, 27
Fractured upper central incisor following trauma, 172
Freeway space, 28, 134, 159
Fremitus, 14
Functional cusp bevel, 29, 125

Gates-Glidden bur, 4
Giant cell arteritis, 160
Gingival overgrowth, 12, 77, 87
Gingivectomy, 87
Gingivitis, 14, 75
Glass ionomer, 20, 24, 52, 99, 101, 103, 119, 126, 156
Glide pathway, 4
Gow-Gates technique, 56
Graft, 79, 85–86, 120
Guide plane, 133, 135
Guided tissue regeneration, 14, 85

Hall technique, 171
Hepatitis B, 155, 157

Ibuprofen, 156
Icon®, 108
Immediate denture, 26, 133
Implants, 120, 171
Index of Orthodontic Treatment Need (IOTN), 42
Indirect retention in denture design, 130
Initial phase of periodontal therapy, 12
International Caries Detection and Assessment System (ICDAS), 103

Kennedy classification, 28, 133
K-flex file, 56
Kidney (renal) disease, 33, 58, 154–155

Laser fluorescence, 98
Lateral condylar inclination (or Bennett angle), 131
Ledermix, 57, 172
Lichen planus, 78, 86
Lichenoid mucosal reactions, 156
Liver disease, 155, 159
Local anaesthetic, 5, 33, 154, 159, 171–172
Localised aggressive periodontitis, 14, 83, 88

Mandibular movement, 131
Maryland bridge, 127
Metal ceramic crown, 97, 122–124
Metronidazole, 57, 76
Midazolam, 33–34
Miller index, 14
Mineral trioxide aggregate, 54, 58
Monostotic fibrous dysplasia, 162

Necrotising ulcerative periodontitis (NUP), 86
Non carious tooth surface loss, 40, 118

Occlusal trauma, 13, 25, 28
Occlusion, 13, 26, 102, 123, 131–133, 154
Odontome, 36
Overdenture, 25

Paget's disease, 58, 161
Partial denture, 25, 27–28, 128–130, 133, 135
Paterson-Kelly (or Plummer-Vinson) syndrome, 161
Penicillin, 35
Peri-implant disease, 119–120, 171
Periodontal probing, 11, 75, 78, 82, 84, 124
Piezograph, 134
Pins, 21, 99, 102
Plaque, 12–14, 19–20, 40, 42, 75, 77–78, 83–87, 119, 124, 160
Post crown, 119
Post-operative sensitivity, 100, 107

Preparation taper, 123
Preventive resin restoration, 20
Primary herpetic gingivostomatitis,
    85
Pulp capping technique, 105–106
Pulpotomy, 41, 97

Quantitative laser fluorescence, 98

Ramsay-Hunt syndrome, 159
Rest seats for partial dentures, 130
Retainer, 26
Retraction cord, 13
Retruded jaw relationship, 26, 29,
    134
Root canal irrigant, 53
Root perforation, 4, 55
Root resorption, 5, 58, 97
Rotary files, 52, 55, 57
RPI (rest, proximal plate, I bar)
    retainer, 129

Selective etch technique, 101, 103
Self-etching bonding systems, 102
Serial extractions technique, 42
Shortened dental arch (SDA), 26
Special tray design, 25, 133
Stephan curve, 20

Temporo-mandibular joint (TMJ),
    153–154, 157
Tetracycline, 76, 83, 156
Thermafil® obturation system, 58
Third molar extraction, 36, 160
TNM classification system, 160
Total etch technique, 101
Trigeminal neuralgia, 160
Tunnel restoration technique, 103

Veneer restoration, 122
Vital pulp therapy for primary teeth,
    171
Von Willebrand's disease, 35